The Dr. Formulated Diet

7 Fat Loss Facts After 40 + 5 Fast Flat Belly Facts

Dr. Amanda Borre, D.C.

© **Copyright 2023 - All rights reserved.**

The content contained within this book may not be reproduced, duplicated or transmitted without direct written permission from the author or the publisher.

Under no circumstances will any blame or legal responsibility be held against the publisher, or author, for any damages, reparation, or monetary loss due to the information contained within this book, either directly or indirectly.

Legal Notice:

This book is copyright protected. It is only for personal use. You cannot amend, distribute, sell, use, quote or paraphrase any part, or the content within this book, without the consent of the author or publisher.

Disclaimer Notice:

Please note the information contained within this document is for educational and entertainment purposes only. All effort has been executed to present accurate, up to date, reliable, complete information. No warranties of any kind are declared or implied. Readers acknowledge that the author is not engaged in the rendering of legal, financial, medical or professional advice. The content within this book has been derived from various sources. Please consult a licensed professional before attempting any techniques outlined in this book.

By reading this document, the reader agrees that under no circumstances is the author responsible for any losses, direct or indirect, that are incurred as a result of the use of the information contained within this document, including, but not limited to, errors, omissions, or inaccuracies.

Table of Contents

A Little Bit About It V

Section 1: 7 Fat Loss Facts After 40 1

Introduction 3

Fact 1: Why Water? 7

Fact 2: Diet Diaries 21

Fact 3: Macros Matter 35

Fact 4: Control Constipation—You Won't See This In The Books For Youngins 59

Fact 5: Everyone Exercise 69

Fact 6: Habits To Hijack 77

Fact 7: Hunger Hacks 101

Conclusion 125

References 129

Section 2: 5 Fast Flat Belly Facts 137

Introduction 139

Chapter 1: Sodium Sensitivity 149

Chapter 2: Embracing Healthy Fats 175

Chapter 3: Managing Gaseous Foods 195

Chapter 4: Food Allergies And Sensitivities 215

Chapter 5: Prioritizing Bowel Regularity 243

Conclusion 269

References 279

A Little Bit About It

My name is Dr. Amanda Borre, D.C., and I'm a mother, daughter, sister, and friend—wearing all of the hats, just like you. I've been helping people become healthier for decades, but the year 2015 was when I really began to zero in on weight-loss issues. I made the switch after seeing that the majority of my overweight female patients were over the age of 40. Now, I'm no stranger to gaining weight and have fought with similar issues in the past, which is why I didn't want the secrets of reducing weight after 40 to be accessible exclusively to those who come to see me in person. In order to provide you with the knowledge in this book, I spent a considerable amount of time doing further research from books, the internet, medical publications, my own personal knowledge, and even my own patients. Because I am patient-obsessed and I enjoy seeing progress, this kind of activity is my absolute passion.

Over the years, I have assisted thousands of people in losing weight, and the reason I have such a high success rate is because I look at each client as an individual and provide them with 1:1 care according to their specific needs. Here, I will be able to give you general knowledge that has worked for the majority of patients. If you want the 1:1 concierge care, just reach out and I would be happy to provide that remotely-anywhere-for you as well. I always try to have an open mind, and I believe I have researched and heard of almost every kind of diet, fad or not, in my clinic. I actually test most anything I hear about myself because I want to give honest feedback when patients ask about other programs. I'd rather test them myself in my clinic because I never want to see any of my patients put their health in danger for a fad diet that might end up doing them more damage in the future. One thing I've learned from all these fad diets is that they don't work in the long run. If you want to lose weight for good, ladies, just keep reading.

Section 1:
7 Fat Loss Facts After 40

Introduction

Ever wonder why those old diet tricks just aren't cutting it anymore? In your 20s and 30s, you could skip a meal here or there or put in some extra time at the gym, and the weight came right off—but not anymore! This is due to the fact that maintaining a healthy weight is harder for our bodies as we get older. This irritating problem affects most women, if not all. You may have seen actress Charlize Theron's recent portrayal of infamous serial murderer Aileen Wuornos in the movie, *Monsters*, or if not, you probably at least know who she is. This amazing actress has a history of changing her physical appearance to play different roles, as shown in *Monsters*, but for her role in another of her greats, *Tully* she really upped the ante. Theron portrays Marlo, a lady who is about to give birth to her third child and is also at risk of developing postpartum depression. This is, however, before her brother sends her an evening nanny called Tully to assist her. Therefore, the usually gorgeous and athletic Charlize Theron—who in real life is a loving mother of two children via adoption—had to put on 50 pounds in order to represent a postnatal figure that was really authentic. Despite the fact that in the past she could more readily put on weight and take it off for previous movie roles, Theron, who was 42 at the time, noted that losing the weight she put on for the role took a lot longer at that age, than it did when she was in her twenties. "Losing that weight took me a year and a half," she said in an interview with (Garcia-Navarro, 2018). "Women do this every day, yet it was one of the worst things my body went through." And she is right; the challenges that women encounter every day do not get nearly enough attention.

Being at this stage can be extremely stressful. It's easy to wonder why your body is suddenly not functioning as it once did. To make things worse, it's also easy to get overwhelmed with different programs that make weight loss promises, leaving you even more perplexed about the best course of action. Are you sick and tired of all the information and just want to know a simple, fast, and well-proven strategy to reduce weight right now? Trust me, I understand; not only as a woman who has researched this topic avidly for quite some time but also as one who has struggled myself, I can confidently state that you've chosen the proper book! In it, I explain why it's more difficult for women over 40 to lose weight and keep it off, as well as how to solve this and lose weight in under a week. I know it seems a bit far-fetched at first, but I promise it will make a lot more sense as you read on.

Why This Is the Right Book for You

Many women find it much more difficult to lose weight once they reach the age of 40 and are perplexed as to why. All of a sudden, the weight-loss strategies they had relied on in the past stopped working. I understand because I've treated a lot of patients like this; in fact, before I discovered the best approach for me and my patients, I went through the same experience. Our bodies change as we age due to a variety of factors, including hormones, stress, and muscle loss, which leads to the accumulation of fat (especially around our belly area). Because of this, I've compiled the most crucial knowledge that will not only show you how to lose weight and keep it off but also lend some answers as to why. After all, it's impossible to begin addressing your weight and health problems after you hit 40 unless you have a firm grasp on the ways in which your body has changed. This book is not about magic cures or fast remedies since, surprise! There are none. If you are serious about losing weight and keeping it off, you will need to put in some effort, but that does not always mean working harder. I will demonstrate how you can work more efficiently to get the results you want in half the time. Imagine if there was a book that showed you how to lose weight without having to do hours of aerobics every day and without always feeling hungry. Well, you're in luck then, because you've just picked up such a book!

Here we go into detail on how water may be your greatest friend when it comes to having glowing skin and rapid weight loss, how your habits can cause you to gain weight unknowingly and what you can do to stop it, how to get rid of constipation and so much more! I've been accused of being too optimistic (and this book will undoubtedly reflect that), but I don't know how else to be after witnessing the outcomes my patients and I have had after following the advice I provide in the following facts. No matter how unsuccessful your previous efforts at weight loss have been, chances are they just weren't the right match for you, or maybe you weren't provided with enough information. In any case, being a Debbie downer won't help you much. Instead, I think that if you remain upbeat and keep trying, you'll eventually succeed. Add to that a realistic plan, and that weight could start coming off in less than a week. Even though we can't stop getting older and it's just a natural part of life, we don't have to "feel" old. Self-confidence is important at any age, and making yourself appear the way you want to is a great place to start. I'm a straightforward gal who thinks that good advice should be useful, instructive, and easy to implement. With the help of this book, you can start right now to look and feel better, lose weight more quickly, and improve your overall health.

Fact 1:

Why Water?

We all know that the saying "Water is life" is more than just a cliche. Besides helping us stay alive, this "drink of life" can actually help us on our weight-loss journey if we're willing to make it our new best friend. While I can't guarantee that chugging a glass of water before bed will cause you to magically lose weight the next morning, there is evidence to suggest that it may help. Water is necessary for every bodily function, which should come as no surprise given that it makes up approximately 60% of the human body. According to research, the more hydrated you are when engaging in tasks like thinking and fat burning, the better your body will perform. For the sake of your general health, it's crucial that you drink enough water each day. By drinking enough water, you may avoid being dehydrated, which can hurt your memory, change your mood, make your body overheat, and cause constipation and kidney stones. Water also has no calories, so drinking it instead of drinks with calories, like sweet tea or sugary soda, can help you control your weight and eat less.

Why Increasing Your Water Intake Aids in Weight Loss:

1. **Water has the ability to naturally reduce your hunger**

   When hunger strikes, your first inclination may be to go for food, but this isn't always the smartest move -or what your body needs. The brain often misinterprets thirst, which is caused by even moderate dehydration, such as hunger. This means that if you are low in water, not food, drinking water may help you feel full. This is why drinking water right before your meal may help you eat less as well. Just think about it for a minute. If, say, drinking two glasses of water makes you feel full, then you will naturally eat less because you are less hungry. (Corney et al., 2015) showed in a small 2015 study that individuals who drank two glasses of water just before a meal ate 22% less than those who did not drink any water before eating. Two glasses of water should be enough to fill your stomach until your brain recognizes fullness. (Davy et al., 2008) performed another trial in which middle-aged overweight and obese volunteers lost 44% more weight when they drank water before each meal than when they did not. The same study also found that drinking water before breakfast cut the number of calories consumed. It's important to note that research on younger people hasn't shown the same dramatic drop in calorie consumption, but middle-aged and older people may benefit a lot more from this.

2. Water May Help to Boost Your Metabolism

Drinking water may help your body burn more calories and speed up its metabolism, which can help you control your weight. In fact, to prove this, a study published by (Vij, 2013) in The Journal of Clinical and Diagnostic Research found that the body mass index and body composition scores of 50 overweight women went down when they drank two cups of water half an hour before each meal for eight weeks. The study's objective was to determine if excessive water consumption helped overweight participants lose weight and body fat. At its conclusion, the research essentially acknowledged and showed the significance of water-induced thermogenesis for the weight loss of obese individuals. Burning calories, or thermogenesis, is a metabolic process that organisms use to create heat. In other words, thermogenesis is the process through which the body "burns" calories to produce heat.

This is not a feat of magic: Water, particularly cold water, seems to boost thermogenesis in the human body. The body must use energy to get the fluid to body temperature; the more energy you burn, the faster your metabolism (the system through which your body converts food and liquids into energy) functions. In a tiny study by

(Boschmann et al., 2003) 14 healthy people drank two cups of 71°F water, and their metabolism increased by 30% on average. Before you fill your glass and still over-pile your plate, you should know that the benefits of thermogenesis probably won't cause you to burn a LOT of calories and lose weight. Because drinking more water has few, if any, negative consequences, it is still important to stay hydrated-even if the impact is minor.

3. **Drinking More Water Can Help You Consume Fewer Liquid Calories Overall**

Because water does not have any calories, drinking it instead of other higher-calorie options like juice, soda, sweetened tea or coffee is one way to cut down on the total number of calories you consume via liquids. Drinking water instead of the typical 20-ounce soft drink from the vending machine can save you 250 calories. The calorie savings may build up rapidly as long as you don't "make up" for those calories, i.e., leave the coffee shop with a bagel and water instead of your typical flavored cappuccino. It's also important to note that although diet soda has no calories, switching to water instead of diet drinks will still help some individuals lose weight. In a study by (Madjd et al., 2015) overweight and obese women who switched from diet drinks to water after their main meal lost more weight while on a weight-loss program. The greater weight reduction in individuals who drank water might be linked to ingesting fewer calories and carbs, according to the researchers, but further study is required.

4. Hydration Is Especially Important While Working Out

During exercise, the body needs water because it dissolves and distributes electrolytes, which are minerals like sodium, potassium, and magnesium that cause the muscles to contract in order to move the body. One of the signs of an electrolyte imbalance, which can happen if you don't drink enough, is cramping. You won't get as much out of your exercises if you don't drink enough water before and throughout your workouts since dehydrated muscle cells break down protein (muscle) more rapidly and develop muscle slower.

During exercise, the body also loses fluids more quickly because it generates heat. This heat is transferred to the surface of the skin, where sweating and evaporation, a cooling process, help keep the body at a comfortable temperature. Maintaining a healthy level of hydration helps keep your blood volume steady, which in turn lets your blood vessels at the surface of your skin expand as much as possible, which helps release heat. If your body can't get rid of too much heat through sweating, you could get heat exhaustion. Hydration may help you get more out of your workout and even your day overall, whether it's by keeping you alert or by helping you stay active for longer. Rather than waiting until you're thirsty, it's important to drink water before, during, and after your workout.

5. **Water Helps Get Rid of Body Waste**

Because water makes up a large portion of urine and because water keeps stools soft, drinking water makes it easier to produce urine and move your bowels. So, if you drink enough water, your digestive system will have an easier time moving things along, and you won't have to worry as much about gas and constipation. Keeping yourself hydrated is also important for maintaining healthy kidney function, getting rid of any germs that may have settled in your urinary system, and avoiding the formation of kidney stones due to too concentrated urine.

6. **Hydration helps boost and sharpen attention**

Fatigue, dizziness, and disorientation are all indicators of dehydration, and who makes good choices when they're feeling like that? Certainly not me! Sleepiness and decreased attentiveness may also be caused by dehydration. Dehydration boosts your body's production of cortisol, the stress hormone. According to a research study published by (Castro-Sepulveda et al., 2018), if you experience any of these symptoms, it may be time to increase your water intake and make some healthier eating choices.

7. **For the body to burn fat, it needs water**

If you don't drink enough water, your body may have a hard time breaking down your stored fat and carbohydrates. This is due to the fact that dehydration results in a decrease in lipolysis inside the body. Lipolysis, which may be brought on by hormonal changes, is the process of breaking down fat to provide energy for the body. (Thornton, 2016) describes how an increase in lipolysis resulted in more weight loss for his subjects in a blog post. Because of this, it is essential to consume an adequate amount of water if you really want to rid your body of the fat that you eat as well as the fat that you store. Not to mention, you also burn more calories at rest when you drink water. This is called resting energy expenditure. Within 10 minutes of consuming water, humans have a 24-30% spike in their resting energy expenditure, which should last for at least an hour. In support of this, research conducted on overweight and obese children and published by (Brown et al., 2006) indicated that their REE increased by 25% after drinking cold water.

In yet another study, participants who were overweight women were asked to increase their water intake to more than one liter (or 34 ounces) each day. The purpose of this study was to explore the consequences of doing so. Also (Stookey et al., 2008) found that this led to an additional loss of 2 kilograms (4.4 lbs) in body weight over the course of a year. These results are very astounding given that the only change these women made to their daily routine was to drink more water. The participants in each study also discovered that drinking 0.5 liters (17 oz) of water resulted in an extra 23 calories burned. That's enough to make you gain more than 2 kilograms (4.4 pounds) of fat in a year, which is about 17,000 calories. When the water is cold, your body expends even more calories in order to warm it up to body temperature, so the colder it is, the better!

8. Becoming Hydrated and Slim—How Much Water Should You Drink?

Imagine being on the best diet for weight loss and still not being able to lose weight fast enough. My buddy Claire experienced this. Even though Claire was exercising four times a week and eating healthily, she was still losing much less weight than she had anticipated in the time frame she had set for herself. She was starting to lose motivation and didn't believe she would ever get to her ideal weight. She admitted to me that she had even considered stopping her morning runs since she often felt lightheaded and disoriented when she tried to push herself over greater distances. The fact that she was a mother to two young boys who kept her rather busy added an extra challenge.

After listening to her, I asked her if she was drinking enough water because she couldn't figure out what she was doing wrong. Yes, she said quickly, but when she thought about it more, she had to admit that her water use had been very random. She said, "I don't always remember to drink water during the day; sometimes I simply drink my coffee." I could absolutely believe it, being a busy mom myself. We often just don't take the time to take care of ourselves or assess simple things like drinking water as a measure of self-care. I explained that because our bodies are mostly water, they need proper hydration to truly thrive. She began to realize that even if she ate the "perfect" diet, she wouldn't lose weight because dehydration makes it impossible for the body to burn fat. But first and foremost, what does it even mean to say that someone is "fully hydrated"? Well, a daily intake of eight 8-ounce glasses of water (or roughly 2 liters) is what is recommended by most health experts. This number is, however, absolutely arbitrary.

The amount of water an individual needs to drink, like so many other things, is totally dependent on the person. Those who are very active, for example, may require more water than those who are not. It is also critical for older people and nursing mothers to monitor their fluid intake. As a general guideline, strive to drink between 0.5 and 1 ounce of water per pound of body weight every day. The basic rule for calculating this is to split your body weight in half. So, if you weigh 200 pounds and do exercise that isn't too hard, you should drink 100 ounces of water. If you want to exercise or go on a track, you should add to those 100 ounces. You should drink 12 ounces of water two hours before your workout and another 12 ounces 30 minutes before it starts. Of course, you should drink during the activities. When figuring out how much water you should consume, you may also want to think about your environment and any illnesses or health problems you have. When it's hot or humid outdoors, you will sweat more and thus need to drink more water. If you are sick, vomiting, or have a fever, you will lose fluid more quickly and will need to rehydrate.

Get a Fun, Pretty Cup So You Like It

Okay, so you know by now that drinking water is basically a necessity if you want to lose weight, but I know that sometimes it can be really hard to consume the recommended 1/2 oz per 1lb of body weight daily. It's very easy to get caught up in your day and forget to drink enough water, which is why carrying a reusable water bottle is always a smart idea. It's much more convenient to have a refillable water bottle on hand when you're out and about, on the road, at your desk, at home, or at your children's school. A water bottle may also act as a sort of visual reminder for you to drink more water if it is kept nearby. Try leaving the bottle on your work desk or anywhere where you spend a lot of time. This continual visual cue will encourage you to drink more water.

Many popular dietitians and coaches who help people lose weight recommend this refillable water method! In fact, registered dietitian Monica Auslander said that carrying water makes you drink more because of the exposure effect (Quinn, 2016). As a psychological phenomenon, the "mere-exposure effect" describes how individuals like something just because they are used to seeing it. It also goes by the name of the "familiarity principle" because of this. Another bonus to this is that the planet will thank you since reusable bottles are also more eco-friendly than using plastic water bottles, which can only be used once. Carrying and using a water bottle that can be used more than once also demonstrates that you are conscientious about the environment and that you are an astute shopper.

One fun way to get more water is to customize your water bottle as you like, which is great for displaying your individuality and creating a fashion statement everywhere you go. What I'm about to say may seem completely out there, but I've found that having a nice water bottle or cup to sip from makes me more likely to keep up with my water intake and push myself a little farther during workouts. And I'm not alone in feeling this way. We all know that humans are drawn to visually beautiful objects, so if you're going to be lugging around a water bottle all day, it might as well be one you like looking at. I guess knowing that our water bottle looks good and makes us look good gives us a little extra motivation, and who doesn't want to look good?

Use a Straw for Easy Access

Straws have been used by humans for thousands of years. The straw has been around since at least 3000 B.C., but at that time, Sumerians used gold tubes to sip on their beers. In the 1800s, straws were made out of rye stalks. Even though the paper straw was invented in 1888, most people didn't start using plastic straws until the 1970s. Straws are commonly used nowadays. Every day, between 170 million and 490 million plastic straws are used in the United States alone. Reusable straws come with most Starbucks or Yeti cups or can be purchased cheaply to go with any mug, tumbler, or cup. They wash easily and are easier on the environment too! Straws also make it easier for those with impairments to drink beverages safely.

However, another benefit you might be surprised to hear about is that straws are actually better for increasing hydration than drinking straight from a cup or bottle. I think most people would expect the reverse, but for some reason, using a straw allows you to consume more water in a shorter period of time. Specialists themselves aren't quite sure why we drink more fluids when we use a straw, but one potential reason is that because it's easier to drink with a straw, we drink more without even realizing it. Straws make it possible to stay hydrated when working on the computer or reading a book without always having to remove the lid. It helps you do more than one thing at once, and it can become a habit that you do without thinking.

I tried this for myself; for two weeks, I sipped all my beverages with a straw. I was surprised to discover that I had consumed more water than usual. I also got similar stories from my patients. Straws aren't for everyone, but I think you'd benefit from giving them a try for a week or so and seeing how you like them. If you're still not convinced, try drinking from a bottle or cup without a straw and then from one with a straw to see if you notice a difference. Be careful when you decide to use a straw with all your drinks because if you're sipping on a high-sugar beverage, it can be easy to gain unwanted weight.

Also, be careful with alcoholic beverages since you might become drunk without even meaning to.

Fact 2:

Diet Diaries

Though it's true that drinking water can help you limit your food intake, it won't do you much good if you're still eating too much or the wrong sorts of food, even if you're drinking enough water. You'll probably not reach your weight-loss goals as fast as you'd like, if at all, depending on what you eat. That's where a food diary can be handy. A food diary allows you to keep track of what you eat and how much you eat in a day. It's easy to overeat during the day, with mindless snacking, busy schedules, chewing sugary gum, etc. Therefore, a food diary can be a very helpful tool for those who want to start taking charge of their eating habits. Tracking what you eat may shed light on your eating routines and habits and reveal your go-to meals, both healthy and otherwise. Keeping a diary has been shown to be a useful strategy for helping individuals who are trying to lose weight alter their eating and exercise habits. (Hollis et al., 2008) did a study on weight loss that included almost 1,700 people. The study found that those who wrote down what they ate every day lost twice as much weight as those who didn't. The research also showed that the best predictors of weight loss were how often people kept food diaries and how much they received support.

How to Make Food Journaling Work for You

Experts in the field of food journaling agree that accuracy and consistency are two of the most important parts of a good food diary. So, what should you jot down, you ask? The following items belong in any basic food journal:

- How much food do you consume? Make a record of how much food and drink you consume at each meal. Indicate the amount in ounces or ordinary household measures (cups, teaspoons, and tablespoons). It is advisable to measure and weigh your meals to the greatest extent possible. If you are away from home, attempt to approximate the portion as best you can.
- In what location are you eating? Write down every place you consume a meal, whether it's at home, in bed, in your car, on the sidewalk, at a friend's house, or at a restaurant. If you happen to be at a restaurant, for instance, note down the name of the place, what you ordered, and how much of the meal you consumed.
- What did you consume today? Write down everything you ate, how it was prepared (boiled, deep fried, baked, etc.), and what you drank throughout the day. Remember to include any

extra toppings, sauces, condiments, or dressings such as sugar, butter, or tartar sauce.

- What time do you eat? Keeping track of the hours at which you consume food, might assist you in recognizing potentially problematic patterns, such as eating late at night. Keeping track of where you eat, what else you do when eating, and how you feel while eating may help you understand some of your routines and give more information.
- What emotions do you experience when eating? Are you happy, depressed, mad, nervous, lonely, bored, or stressed? By documenting how you feel at certain times, you may identify your triggers.
- With whom are you dining? If you aren't dining alone, who else may be present during your meal? A coworker, spouse, friend? Maybe you eat more when you're with certain people and don't even realize it.
- Do you have any other activities going on when you're eating? Are you interacting with friends or family, watching TV, using your laptop, or viewing something else? In this section, list any activities you do while eating or drinking. This may help you identify if you are a mindless eater and begin working on it.

How to Keep a Good Food Diary

- As soon as you finish the meal or drink, note it down. Avoid waiting until the end of the day since your memory will probably be less precise. Life gets hectic, and it is easy to forget the details if you wait until the end of the day. Therefore, writing it down immediately helps you get a more accurate picture of what you are really eating throughout the day or can help you plan ahead for what you are going to eat that day (which is even better.)

- Don't forget to mention any alcoholic drinks you take. Alcoholic beverages generally have a lot of sugar, so they can add up fast!

- You can help yourself further by using a smartphone app like Lose It! or MyFitnessPal. Calories and other dietary details are also available in these applications.

- When describing the meal or drink, be as descriptive as you can. Take an espresso as an example; when you drink this, pay close attention to the brand and the amount of your beverage. Similarly, after each meal, measure or estimate how much food you ate. Getting a measuring scale to help you weigh how much you're eating may help here.

So, You've Decided to Keep a Record of Everything You Eat. What Now?

Take a step back and review your entries after you've completed a week of food journaling. Look for any recurring tendencies, patterns, or routines; for instance, you may take into consideration items like:

- How nutritious is my diet? Pay close attention if you consume a lot of processed, sugary, or dairy-containing meals. Processed foods, in particular, include high proportions of added sugar, salt, and fat. Although these substances improve the flavor of the food we eat, consuming too much of them could result in major health problems, including obesity, heart disease, diabetes, and other cardiovascular diseases. Because of the extra sugar and fat, these foods also tend to have a higher calorie count. So, if you notice yourself nibbling on potato chips or buying a lot of ready-to-eat meals from the supermarket during the week, it's time to break the habit.

- Do I eat whole grains every day? The health benefits of whole grains are different from those of processed grains, which have been linked to problems like obesity and inflammation. A diet, high in whole grains, has been linked to several health benefits, such as a lower risk of diabetes, heart disease, and high blood pressure. Products created from whole grains are more satisfying than those made from refined grains, and some studies show that eating them may reduce the risk of obesity. A meta-analysis of 15 studies with almost 120,000 people found that eating the recommended three servings of whole grains every day was linked to a lower BMI and less belly fat (Harland & Garton, 2008).

- Do I eat or drink things that have sugar added to them? If yes, how often? The body may get its energy from sugar, a kind of carbohydrate. But long-term sugar consumption can cause weight gain. Sugar is in a lot of foods, both natural ones like fruit and processed ones like mass-produced bread and canned vegetables, not to mention sugary drinks and teas. For most adult women, the American Heart Association (AHA) recommends consuming no more than 100 calories per day (about 6 teaspoons or 24 grams of sugar), whereas, for most adult males, the recommended daily intake is 150 calories (around 9 teaspoons or 36 grams of sugar). Do my feelings have an impact on what I eat? When I'm worried or fatigued, do I find myself craving bad foods? Emotional eaters eat to get through difficult times. Emotional eating is a common phenomenon that affects a lot of people. Eating a bag of chips when sad or a chocolate bar after a challenging day at work are two examples of how it could manifest, but a person's life, health, happiness, and weight can all be hurt by emotional eating if it happens often or if it is the main way they deal with their feelings. When you give in to a yearning for food and eat it, your brain releases a neurotransmitter called dopamine, which makes you feel good. The process of craving something other than food and then fulfilling that craving will give your body the same chemical outcome. If you make a list of new habits to replace eating as a response to good or bad stress, you get the same "high" and a healthier outcome. I cannot create this list for you because you have to crave it. It needs to be something you enjoy that takes about the same amount of time as eating a snack, 2-5 minutes. When you retrain the habit of "stress eating" now, it will make keeping your weight off easier for life. Make this list today. Hand-write it. Put copies in your bathroom, on the refrigerator, in your purse or bag, and in your car. The next time you feel yourself starting to reach for food to cope, do something else on the list and note the feeling you have afterward. Accomplishment! Emotional eating can be caused by a lot of different things, not just bad emotions like stress.

People also say that they are triggered by boredom, exhaustion, social pressures, and unhealthy habits like rewarding themselves with sweet snacks all the time. Luckily, the first step in getting rid of emotional eating is to figure out what makes it happen in your life. Keeping a food journal might help you figure out the circumstances in which you are more prone to eat for emotional reasons than for physical ones.

You may learn more about your own eating patterns by monitoring this activity. How often do I eat while moving? When we're pressed for time, we turn to fast food, freezer meals, and even the closest gas station for quick, practical answers. Our bodies suffer as a result of the bad nourishment that results from this. Eating on the run also means we eat faster, which leads to us eating more. So, if you find that you tend to eat too much when you're in a hurry, work on stopping this habit. When we take the time to enjoy actual meals, our relationship with food changes. But of course, I do understand that life does get busy sometimes, so if you do fast food, almost every drive-through has a salad with grilled chicken, lettuce, and tomato. Gas stations have salads, fruit, or hard-boiled eggs available for quick protein. Don't let a busy schedule become an excuse for you to eat poorly. There are great choices out there. It's up to you to make the right choice in these moments to get the outcome you want-the healthiest you!

Craft Your Own Stylish Notebook

If you would rather not buy a ready-made diary, you can also make a personalized notebook in less than 15 minutes. You only need a few basic supplies and tools.

There are several ways to make notebooks, but this one has been the most reliable and flexible for my needs. In terms of page count and cover content, the sky's the limit (provided that you are able to make holes for the stitching in the cover). Don't overlook the importance of creating a stunning and unique design for the cover. If it looks attractive to your eyes, you will reach for it more often.

First Step—Compile all of your materials. You must first acquire a few tools and materials before you can begin. For equipment, you need a ruler, cutting board, needle, utility knife, sharpening steel, hammer, and leather punch. As for supplies, office paper; and the cover, cardboard, thread, paper, and tape (which is optional). Once you have the necessary equipment and materials, you may begin assembling it.

Second Step—First, Get several pieces of letter-size printer paper, cut them in half, and fold each piece in half. Once everything has been folded over, you will have a 4.25 x 5.5 inches notebook that fits perfectly in your pocket and that is large enough for both taking notes and drawing. Of course, there is no restriction on the size of the notebook; you may build it any way you choose.

Third Step—personalize the cover of your notebook with a sketch, print, or anything else you'd want to use before you sew it together. The possibilities here are almost endless.

Fourth Step—Make holes for sewing.

1. Arrange the pages facing the cover.
2. Mark the areas where the holes will be. Set the holes at a distance of 1 cm from the edge.
3. Use a punch to go through the holes. To do what you need to, you will essentially want a spike that can be struck with a hammer. Use anything that will create a circular hole as much as possible (this will eliminate tearing).

Fifth Step—Put It All Together: Start sewing on the inside of the notebook (at the bottom edge) and leave a short tail of thread to tie a knot at the beginning.

After stitching all the way through, go back to the beginning and tie a knot. Because of this, the binding between the pages and the cover is strong, solid, and long-lasting.

Sixth Step—Paper Tape (optional): You have the option of covering the notebook's spine with paper tape. Even though it's not necessary, this is a great way to finish off the design of a paper notebook.

Seventh Step—Trim the Extra Paper: Trim any extra paper that will protrude from the center of the notebook.

Eighth Step—If this notebook shouts "You!" when you look at it, you're finished. Everything can be altered to suit your preferences, including the size, number of pages, and layout. You will get a creative, practical, and very robust notebook using this technique. This makes for an aesthetically pleasing food journal. If you like the look and feel of it, you will be more likely to enjoy using it.

Measuring Food on the Fly

Portion sizes are important when trying to lose weight, and using a food scale or measuring cup will give you the most accurate results. Nevertheless, pulling out a food scale every time you sit down to eat may not always be a feasible option. So, you will have to make an educated guess about the right size of items sometimes. Fortunately, there are a few strategies you may use to accurately estimate portion sizes. Using your hands as a measuring tool is a quick and easy way to figure out how much food is in different serving sizes. Even if you're dining at a five-star establishment, the fact that it's a part of your body makes it a very practical measurement tool. However, since each person has somewhat different-sized hands, it's best to gain some experience with actual measurements before trying to guess how much something should be. When attempting to determine portion size, use these recommendations:

Protein consumption can be calculated using the palm of your hand. A serving of protein weighing 4 oz. is equal to one palm. Pork, poultry, beef, fish, and chicken are some examples of foods that you may measure a 4 oz. portion of.

A one-cup serving is roughly the size of a cupped hand. Food products like pasta, potatoes, almonds, and even ice cream can all be measured with the use of this tool.

A serving size of one tablespoon is about the same as the very tip of your thumb. Mayonnaise, cheese, salad dressings, creams, and peanut butter are all high in fat; hence, this instrument is used to determine how much of those foods a person consumes.

For measuring carbs, a fist works well. When trying to calculate how much rice, cereal, salad, fruit, or popcorn you've had, use this tool.

One teaspoon of oil or fat is about equal to the size of the thumbnail. Olive oil, butter, and salad dressings may all be measured with this.

Pre-planning and food preparation are keys to success in healthful eating. Sit down once a week when you have a small chunk of time. Look through your social calendar, the food in your fridge, freezer, and pantry, and plan your shopping list. Let the social calendar dictate which meals will be at home and which might be out. If those are home meals, plan the shopping list to use both what you have and buy only what you will need. If those meals will be fast food or restaurants, look at the menus online and determine what you will order. Pre-populate the food journal with your food plan for the week. Write meals in one color ink. For any changes that happen out of your control and do not end up going as planned, write in red. This makes for easy reference later. You can easily see what percentage of your food goes as planned and how many times you veered off the planned course.

The Power of a Good Attitude

I've already said that I'm a huge believer in positive thinking, and with good reason. Positive thinking and successful weight reduction go hand in hand, which shouldn't come as much of a surprise. I've found that keeping an optimistic frame of mind has helped me and my patients very much in our quest to shed pounds. I mean, just think about it, fixating on one's own past failure, and current discontentment makes weight loss difficult if not darn near impossible. And why is this the case? For the simple reason that dwelling on the bad causes us to give in to our desires, consume too much, and neglect our regular workout routine. Negative thinking patterns may hinder our weight reduction attempts in a number of ways, including beating ourselves up every time we consume the wrong foods, becoming preoccupied with what we can't eat, and approaching our workout routine with dread. A bad self-perception makes us feel helpless, unhappy, or uninspired, which increases the likelihood that we'll miss our daily exercise or eat a bag of chips to feel better. But understanding those emotions and changing those ideas into something more uplifting might really assist us in achieving our objectives. Here are some methods for developing a more optimistic outlook:

1. Keep cards with your objectives, motivational pictures, affirmations, and quotes visible.

This keeps us motivated when we'd rather give up and serves as a helpful reminder to adopt an optimistic outlook. Imagine coming home from work absolutely exhausted and without any enthusiasm to exercise. However, seeing pictures of your goals plastered all over your wall would likely spur you on to go for that run won't it? Having something to look at that constantly reminds you that your dreams and goals are valuable is better than having nothing at all.

2. List Three Positive Aspects of Your Day

   These should be items over which you have some measure of influence, such as getting up early to jump some rope before even having breakfast, looking forward to a hot shower after a sweaty workout, or the taste of a chocolate protein shake for breakfast. See how your mood changes after a week of trying it out. The human brain has a natural inclination toward negativity, but this practice may help retrain it to see and appreciate the positive aspects of everyday life.

3. Stop Telling Yourself Bad Things

   If you find yourself having unproductive thoughts, consider replacing them with a string of positive affirmations. There are many books, podcasts, and videos online with endless positive affirmations.

Fact 3:

Macros Matter

Now that you have spent a week writing down and tracking everything as you eat it, and crafted a beautiful, aesthetically pleasing journal, you are ready to take food journaling to the next level. The term "macro" stands for macronutrients. Protein, carbohydrates, and fats are the three major classes of nutrients that make up the majority of the food that you consume and are the primary sources of the majority of the energy that you need. Keeping track of your macros means keeping track of how many grams of protein, carbohydrates, and fat you eat each day. You can make (or prepare to make) more informed, nutritious eating choices if you keep track of your macros.

The idea is similar to counting calories or points, but it goes further than that. Simply put, weight loss does not always occur when the calories burned exceed the calories consumed. Understanding the sources of those calories and how they affect your body is made easier with macro counting. Furthermore, it teaches you that not all calories are created equal. Let's suppose, for illustration purposes, that your daily calorie target is 2,000. Protein has a caloric value of four per gram. Therefore, a 125-gram serving of protein contains 500 calories, leaving 1,500 calories for fat and carbohydrates. Focusing more on the nutritional content of food is always preferable since it helps people pay closer attention to how their bodies are fueled and how their bodies respond. By concentrating on getting enough protein, and fats and paying more attention to the kind of carbs you are consuming rather than just calories alone, you may experience higher satiety (less hunger) and be better able to achieve your fitness goals. Another advantage of macro counting is that it is a versatile strategy. It's called "flexible dieting" because you still eat real food and don't starve your body. The phrase "If It Fits Your Macros," which means you may eat anything as long as it fits into your macros, is often used by those who track their percentage of carbohydrates/proteins/fats.

Should you now manipulate the system so you can consume just donuts? Obviously, no. But is it possible to occasionally indulge in a sweet treat or two and still achieve success? Yes! When you are counting macros, there is no such thing as a "cheat" meal; all that happens is that you have to rearrange some of your macros to make room for the new item. It is indeed possible to shed extra pounds, keep your muscles from wasting away, and keep your appetite in check by counting macros. Reading food labels and diet research out there can be really confusing, so paying attention to just these three categories can be really helpful. Some nutritionists worry that a macronutrient plan oversimplifies the problem and doesn't take into account the mental and social factors that lead to unhealthy eating. Still, some defend the simplicity as beneficial. I believe it is a great place to start. Take into account social/emotional issues as best you can with planning ahead, use the habit replacement tip mentioned earlier in this book, attend overeaters anonymous meetings if you need group support, reach out to mental health counselors when necessary, or you may reach me directly via www.lifelongmetaboliccenter.com if you need 1:1 help. Simplicity can be a beautiful thing, but please do not be too proud or scared to reach out when you need help. That's the blessing of the modern world and our abundant resources.

The Top 3 Best Ways to Use Macros to Lose Weight

Macros are totally conditional upon factors like age, height, and physicality. A person who leads a more sedentary lifestyle will need a lower total daily intake of carbohydrates and a higher total daily intake of protein than, say, an athlete would. For the most part, however, you can use these proportions as a general benchmark:

- If you workout for sixty minutes or less every day: 40% carbohydrates, 30% fat, and 30% protein

- With a daily workout regimen of one to two hours: 45% carbohydrates, 25% fat, and 30% protein

- If your everyday workout exceeds two hours, think about consulting Dr. Borre 1:1. To keep up that high physical output and healthily lose weight, you need customization.

Now that you know what the best macro ratio is, you can figure out how many macros you need and keep track of them in three easy steps:

1. Determine Your Caloric Requirements

    Again, the answer to this question exactly depends on things like your age, size, amount of exercise, and how much weight you want to lose, but a rough estimate would be to add one zero to your ideal body weight. For example: if you want to weigh 140 lbs., you should consume approximately 1400 calories per day.

2. Total the macros you used

    When you know how many calories you should consume each day, you can use your macronutrient ratio to calculate precisely how many grams of protein, fat, and carbohydrates to take in daily. A macro calculator, such as the one from freedieting.com, can help you save time because this requires a bit of calculating on your part. Using this technology, I found that a woman who ate 1,500 calories a day and worked out for 30 minutes most days of the week would need 150 grams of carbs, 112 grams of protein, and 50 grams of fat every day.

2. To Keep Tabs on Your Macros, Download an App Like MyfitnessPal or Use One of Your Beautifully Crafted Journals

You should keep note of the quantities of each macronutrient that you consume at each meal and snack now that you know how much you require. Using a meal tracker app is one efficient method for doing this. Using these numbers, you can pre-plan your week, prep foods ahead of time, and then just work the plan! If the concept of a macro diet as a whole, leaves you feeling overwhelmed, just know that you are not alone in this feeling. There is no doubt that dedication is necessary for this level of meticulous tracking. I understand that it can be especially difficult if you're someone who dines out often. Therefore, I'm suggesting a simpler, but less accurate, way, which is to simply use your eyes. Make a bit more than a quarter of your plate lean protein and around a quarter of your plate whole grains or starchy veggies (like baked potatoes) if you're trying to get your macros in but detest monitoring meals or can't at the moment. You should fill up the rest of your plate with vegetables that don't have starch but are still counted as carbohydrates. You don't have to worry about including fat on your plate if you include foods like salad greens dressed in a vinaigrette or chicken grilled in olive oil that already contains fat. And if it doesn't satisfy your hunger, load up on the green stuff. You won't be able to verify that your macros are in the perfect 30/30/40 range with this strategy, but you will be able to make sure you eat enough protein and avoid consuming too many refined carbohydrates. Also, it will aid you in controlling your portion sizes. In fact, doing both can speed up your progress toward a slimmer physique.

Pay Attention to Your Carb Intake

What would you say if I asked you whether or not you eat a balanced, nutritious diet? Well, assuming you're like the majority of Americans, you'd likely respond, "Heck yes." Approximately 75% of Americans say they don't worry about what they consume because they believe they eat relatively healthily. But this is simply untrue. In fact, according to (Paddock, 2015), a shocking 76% of Americans weren't getting enough fruit, and 87% weren't getting enough vegetables. The fact that the average size of our portions is only becoming larger really isn't helping our obesity problem. As it stands, the percentage of obese people in the United States is now more than 25% in 48 states, 35% in nine states, and 30% in 31 states.

In fact, an investigation of dietary patterns by (Shan et al., 2019) found that Americans consume much more saturated fat and refined carbs than is healthy. The study, which followed 43,996 people from 1999 to 2016, revealed that Americans had gradually reduced their use of "low-quality" carbohydrates, including overly processed grains and sugary snack items. But in absolute terms, the decline is merely 3%. Even so, Americans still don't eat enough of the healthier types of carbs. Whole grains high in fiber, fruits, and vegetables are examples of high-quality carbohydrates. Low-quality carbohydrates make up 42% of the average American diet, whereas high-quality carbs make up just 9%. Not only will these poor carbohydrates likely exacerbate your weight loss troubles, but they may also significantly raise your risk of type 2 diabetes and cardiovascular disease. Especially as we age, our vulnerability to these sorts of things increases. So, don't just think of clean eating as a good way to keep weight off. The wellness of your body depends on it as well.

In contrast to whole grains, processed carbohydrates have all their fiber, vitamins, and minerals removed, making them immediately absorbed by the body upon consumption. Our body's ability to burn fat is abruptly overridden by this, which also causes a sharp rise in blood sugar and the production of large amounts of insulin. Because of this, our body does not utilize the processed carbohydrates we ate as fuel and instead stores them as extra body fat. Having said that, eliminating all carbohydrates from your diet is not always the best course of action, so remember everything is in moderation.

While eliminating ALL carbs may be fruitful for a select few, most people would find it unsatisfying and unsustainable. That is why, after you assess your food diary and understand your daily eating patterns if you are overeating carbs, you need to make a personalized plan on how to gradually reduce your carb intake for your desired goal. If you notice you eat a lot of processed carbs throughout the day like white bread, pasta, white flour, donuts, etc., you should make an active attempt to replace them with higher-quality carbs. If say, for example, you notice from your notebook that you have a tendency to eat a lot of cupcakes when you are watching TV. Well now begin to implement steps to change this habit. You can begin by replacing all those sweet desserts with naturally sweet fruit like apricots or apples. So now every time you find yourself mindlessly eating away at least it'll be fiber-filled goodies. By the end of your show, you'll probably find that you ate less food than usual too. That's better for most because cutting out carbs entirely is unsustainable in the long term.

I see a lot of patients in my clinic who were successful at cutting carbs, but the minute they came back, so did the weight-and it brought friends. Fiber's presence in food can slow digestion in the stomach, helping you feel fuller for longer. Also, high-fiber foods are low in calories, which makes for a good strategy. Want the best news ever? You can actually eat carbs every day without having to worry about getting fat. People mistake all carbohydrates as being the same and having the same effect on the body. It's actually complex carbs that support our ideal well-being, while simple processed carbohydrates are what essentially causes weight gain. Simple carbs have the same addictive qualities as sugar and therefore are also easy to grow hooked on.

The brain's reward circuitry is profoundly affected by them. Dopamine, which is responsible for emotions like pleasure and reward, is released when we eat carbohydrates. When you eat processed carbohydrates, your brain responds by generating a lot of dopamine almost instantaneously. This feel-good moment is what makes people want to continue eating. If ingested to an excessive degree and on a frequent basis, this will cause the brain to get used to it, at which point it will "require" simple carbohydrates in order to feel satisfied. And so starts the addictive loop. That explains in part why so many Americans consume so many processed foods without giving them a second thought.

As I indicated before, the answer isn't to eliminate all carbohydrates; rather, it's to swap them out for more complex ones and usually reduce the amount. Complex carbohydrates are digested quite differently from simple carbs, despite the fact that they also convert to sugar in the body. Due to their high fiber, vitamin, and mineral content, which enters the system more gradually, complex carbohydrates help slow down digestion and maintain healthy blood sugar levels. After incorporating them into your regular diet, you won't feel dependent on unhealthy foods anymore since it doesn't significantly raise your blood sugar, release high quantities of the hormone that stores fat in your body, or secrete dopamine in the brain. Examples of processed carbohydrates are anything that has been man-made like cereal, tortillas, bread, or pasta. Simple carbohydrates are those that come from the earth like rice, potatoes, yams, couscous, or zucchini.

What Is a Micronutrient?

While the phrase "macronutrients" refers to proteins, lipids, and carbs, the term "micronutrients" refers to vitamins and minerals. Generally speaking, your body cannot create vitamins and minerals; thus, humans must get their micronutrients from the diet. They are also known as vital nutrients because of this. Vitamins are created by plants and animals and are susceptible to decomposition when exposed to high temperatures, acids, or air. Contrarily, minerals are inorganic, found in either soil or water, and are not decomposable under normal conditions. Whenever you eat, you take in the minerals and vitamins that the food you ate originally had.

To ensure that you are getting adequate vitamins and minerals, it is better to consume a range of meals since each item has varied amounts of micronutrients. Since each vitamin and mineral has a distinct purpose in your body, an appropriate intake of all micronutrients is essential for achieving maximum health. Vitamins and minerals are necessary for normal development, immune system function, brain maturation, and many other vital activities. Some micronutrients, depending on how they are used, can also aid in the prevention and treatment of certain illnesses. One potential reason for weight gain is micronutrient insufficiency. A balanced diet is SO important for good health, and that includes both Macro and Micronutrients in sufficient quantities. Four hot ones right now are:

Calcium

Although best known for strengthening bones and teeth, calcium also aids in maintaining a healthy weight. There are studies out there that demonstrate calcium consumption can truly help you lose weight, so do not cut these out entirely. Moderation again is key. I have personally seen these results with my own patients. It's important to note that when you cut down on your calorie intake generally, meals high in calcium are proven to help you lose weight.

Potassium

Potassium, a little-spoken-of micronutrient, is a vitamin that is helpful for weight reduction and is essential for helping muscles recover after exercise. Additionally, it aids in the body's detoxification process and may lessen bloating by eliminating too much salt. Both the heart and the kidneys benefit from potassium's presence. Bananas, mushrooms, spinach, and sweet potatoes, are all good sources of potassium.

Fats in omega-3

Two health advantages of eating foods high in omega-3 fatty acids are a healthier heart and skin. As an added bonus, it may help you lose weight by making you feel fuller for longer. Metabolic rate and the number of calories burned during exercise may both increase from supplementation with omega-3 fatty acids. Walnuts, soybeans, canola oil, chia seeds, and fatty fish like salmon, sardines, and tuna are examples of foods high in omega-3 fatty acids.

Magnesium

With the help of this micronutrient, bloating, and water retention can be minimized, and blood flow enhanced. In those who are overweight or obese, magnesium may control insulin levels and, therefore, blood sugar levels. The mineral magnesium may be found in abundance in foods like beans, nuts, and seeds, as well as in green, leafy vegetables.

Shelly's Story-When Keto Isn't All Bad

After being told that he had cancer, my friend Jeff, husband and father of three boys, chose to follow the ketogenic diet over chemotherapy and conventional methods of treatment. The popularity of the keto diet is unprecedented. The keto diet is so popular that many dieters credit it for their success in losing weight-plus the fact that it is extensively promoted by so many celebrities and fitness "gurus" on Instagram.

Shelly, his wife, decided she would do it with him along with their whole family. They had MAJOR motivation to follow it to the letter and long term. He was given a short prognosis for life expectancy. Jeff believes that despite doctors saying his tumor was incurable, it shrank as a result of his diet, which comprises very little to no carbs. Almost no surgeon would even consider operating on it. After a period of time, one surgeon was able to successfully remove a portion of it. When you have cancer, diagnostic testing utilizes sugar for imaging because it goes directly to "feed" cancer, therefore making it easy to visualize. Doesn't it make sense that we wouldn't want to feed cancer? Shelly lost weight and felt amazing. Jeff went on to be the longest-living person on record at the time of his type of cancer. Although a few studies have shown it could be able to treat specific cancers, the diet is not one that is often advised by doctors for the prevention or treatment of cancer, and I'm not sure why, so talk to your doctor if this is a concern for you or a family member. Another potential reason why the diet may help treat tumors is that it has the potential to inhibit tumor development, safeguard healthy cells, reduce inflammation, and enhance the efficacy of anti-cancer medications. Use common sense, consult your doctor, and make educated decisions based on what makes the most sense for you, but overall, very low-carb diets are tough to sustain unless you are highly motivated to do it forever.

There are a lot of articles about the diet online, and stores carry a wide range of foods that are good for people who are on it. Even many of my own patients want to give it a try and often ask me how to get started. The ketogenic diet, or "keto" for short, entails eating very little carbohydrates and a high-fat diet. When you eat a low-carbohydrate ketogenic diet, your body quickly burns up the carbs stored in your muscles and liver as glycogen. You switch to burning fat after your glycogen reserves are exhausted. During this phase, many individuals see significant weight reduction, which is why so many other people are eager to give it a try.

Why to NOT Keto

However, despite these assertions and interests, the majority of health care providers, including physicians and nutritionists, do not advocate for it. The ketogenic diet is not something I recommend to my patients since I am not a fan of it myself. First of all, it's not a healthy approach to maintain weight loss, and I know this from personal experience since practically every patient I've treated who had been on the keto diet gained the weight back as soon as they quit the diet. This was the case with American actress, producer, and fitness expert Tamra

Judge. The Glendale, California-born reality personality has a history of experimenting with new diets and exercise routines, and in June 2021 she stated that she would be trying the ketogenic diet (Berg, 2021). Although Tamara is renowned for her diet-related open-mindedness, she wasn't a fan of the keto diet before attempting it because of all the health risks, but she gave it a try nonetheless in the hopes that it might help with her autoimmune difficulties.

A couple of months after beginning the diet, one of her Instagram followers asked whether she was still following the low-carb plan; she responded, "No, I put on weight while on Keto," with a sad emoji. Nutritionists aren't fans for a variety of reasons, not only long-term maintenance. The lack of fruits and whole grains on the ketogenic diet makes me dislike it even more since I know that it might induce constipation in certain people. Constipation is a miserable condition in and of itself, but anybody who has suffered from it knows that if it persists for an extended period of time, it may also cause hemorrhoids and rectal tears. Plus, while you're out and about with the family and kids, the last thing you want to do is spend a long time in the restroom because of constipation. On the ketogenic diet, you can't eat a lot of starchy vegetables, lentils, or yogurt. This makes you more likely to be malnourished. It may also raise your risk of heart disease due to its high saturated fat content. The keto diet's exclusion of whole foods groups long term is a big turn-off for my scientific brain. The rigor of the diet is a problem as well. It's very difficult for a single person to follow a lifestyle that calls for so many sacrifices, such as calculating carbs, cutting out whole food categories, monitoring protein consumption, and limiting food options within authorized groups., but to keep these limitations in place over time is extremely unlikely for anybody. Parents who are attempting to set a positive example for their children in regard to diet and nutrition want to follow guidelines that appear healthy and well-balanced.

How to NOT Keto

As you may have gathered from my above text, I am not a proponent of the keto diet. I have seen far too many patients come to me after doing it short term only to have acquired more weight in a short time afterward. That being said, I do believe there is oodles of research out there about the typical American diet and culturally how excessive our "normal" carb intake is. So even though I won't tell you to go "no carb" or "low carb", what you may need is likely less than you think is normal now. For exact numbers on macro counts for your body, you may contact me directly at www.lifelongmetaboliccenter.com.

How to Exercise After 40 to Lose Fat and Gain Muscle

No matter what program you choose, the six things below should be the most important parts of your workout routine if you want to gain lean muscle mass, become more physically active, and look better after 40.

Always Warm Up

The warm-up phase of our exercise regimen becomes more crucial as we age. The last thing you want is to be hurt and unable to get in your weekly workouts, play with your children, or go to work. Also, as we get older, our bodies tend to lose some of their flexibility. Therefore, warming up is essential if you want to continue exercising regularly in the future, and it's also crucial to prevent injuries. Warm up thoroughly, and pay specific attention to your shoulders, hips, ankles, and knees. A nice place to start is with some dynamic stretches and a little mild cardio. Just always keep in mind that you're trying to prevent injuries because they can really hold you back from attaining your goals. It may take more time than in the past to bounce back from a setback as well, so it's best to avoid them if possible.

Weekly Weight Lifting

It's possible that you won't be able to lift weights four times a week like you used to. Perhaps due to time or perhaps body restrictions. Yet, if you want to gain muscle, lifting is a great way to trigger the growth response necessary. Exercises that train many muscle groups and joints at once, such as squats, deadlifts, bench presses, and cleans, are the greatest for increasing strength. Lifting two or three times per week, 3 sets, with around 8–15 repetitions per set, is a tried-and-true strength training regimen for gaining muscle beyond 40. (Warmup sets are recommended before attempting these.) To maximize improvement, keep your routine simple and make little weight increases per week. But if you're a beginner, you should definitely start with lower weights to avoid injury. You may get discomfort in some body parts, such as the wrists, elbows, and so on, but you should not have PAIN. You can lift more weight by using complex movements in combination with these rep schemes, which will result in a bigger metabolic reaction.

Workout With Cardio Several Times Each Week

Weightlifting is fantastic, but for optimal results, you must also do some cardiovascular exercise. When we do 30–40 minutes of cardiovascular activity, it helps to boost our metabolism for the next 24 hours. In addition to jogging (or fast walking if you're new to it), jumping rope, swimming, burpees, squat jumps, and cycling, you might also practice other exercises that you find enjoyable that raise your heart rate and break a sweat.

Rest, Rest, Rest

If you want to gain muscle beyond the age of 40, sleep is a necessity. The body overflows with feel-good chemicals that encourage recuperation and repair when we are sleeping. (Not just skeletal muscles, but also the nervous system and internal organs.) If you aren't getting enough shut-eye, it may be one of the factors adding to your weight gain. Getting a good night's sleep is another way to boost your strength at the gym. Your exercise routine can deteriorate if you don't receive enough of it. As you get older, you may find it harder to get enough sleep due to work, children, and other factors in your life. But it should be one of your top concerns if you don't want to gain weight or do want to keep your muscles from getting smaller. And by that, I don't simply mean getting more sleep but also making sure that the sleep you do receive is good sleep. Sleep in a dark room, consistently as opposed to broken sleep/naps, no tech before bed. These can all increase the quality of your sleep.

Power Proteins

Protein is the nutritional building block for growing lean muscle. After 40, protein needs to be given even more attention than in our younger days. When you are between the ages of 40 and 50, your protein demands rise to roughly 1-1.2 grams per kilogram, or 75–90 grams per day for a 75-kilogram individual (Wempen, 2022). Regular exercisers also have greater requirements, ranging from 1.1 to 1.5 grams per kilogram. 1.2–1.7 grams per kilogram are required for those who routinely lift weights or are preparing for a race.

Get Your Supplements

Some supplements can be really helpful in your muscle-gaining mission. Though do Understand that supplements are just the "extra 10%" that get you where you need to go. They don't take the place of a disciplined workout regimen or a healthy diet. To assist you in muscle building, consider the following:

- Fish oil may help you exercise and lift more frequently by lowering inflammation.
- Whey protein: Nutritional supplementation with whey protein powder after exercise has been shown to hasten recovery. Protein shakes like Quest, or Fairlife Elite can be easy, portable ways to get more delicious protein in your life.
- BCAA's-Branch Chain Amino Acids are a great way to hasten muscle recovery after your workout. Most have great fruity flavors and feel y much like a post-workout treat.

Myths Surrounding the Keto Diet

Myth #1: When on keto, you are continually burning fat

So, you already know that the key "benefit" of the ketogenic diet is that it puts your body into a state known as "fat-burning mode." You've switched from using sugar as an energy source to using fat as fuel 24/7. And to be fair, this is correct. Ketosis refers to the condition in which your body begins to burn fat. That being said, even if your body is in ketosis, you primarily burn food fat before any stored body fat. Always being in a state of ketosis does not guarantee weight loss. To ensure success, you still have to be in a calorie deficit, stay there for an extended period of time, and not break your fast with garbage food.

Myth #2: When Eating Keto, You Don't Need to Track Your Calories.

Some advocates of the ketogenic diet claim that, once in ketosis, calories no longer count and that you may eat as much butter and bacon as you want without gaining weight. This is such an annoying myth for me, especially when you think about how important the quality of foods is whether or not you're trying to lose weight. Calorie deficit is easy to understand. You burn off a certain amount of calories each day. If you eat more calories than you exert, you will gain weight. And you'll lose weight if you consume fewer calories than you expend. Simple as that. Pair this with eating the right ratio of carb/fat/protein per day, and you've got a winner. You can't tell me eating bacon and butter in excess truly makes sense for good health, right?

Myth #3: Everyone Has Equal Carbohydrate Needs

Your own body will determine how many carbs you should consume-not a generic restriction number and definitely not ZERO. When first beginning a ketogenic or other extremely low-carb diets, it is easy to underestimate the extent to which your diet will restrict carbohydrate intake. Well, in order to assist the body in entering ketosis, followers often start on the lower end of the 20–50 gram range of carbs per day. But of course, with some tweaks (such as increasing your exercise), you may be able to push intake further. Those who have trouble using fat as fuel due to genetics may find it very challenging, if not impossible to lose weight by using this dieting method.

Myth #4: There's No Such Thing as Too Much Protein

Although low in carbohydrates, it is not the same as the Atkins Diet. A breakfast of eggs and smoked salmon and a supper of steak may seem delicious, but protein should be consumed in proportion with other nutrients. This is one distinction between the ketogenic and the Atkins diets. Any more protein than your body needs may be turned into glucose, which can cause a spike in blood sugar. Furthermore, a keto dieter who already has high amounts of ketones in their body may have problems due to the breakdown of amino acids in the protein, which may result in an increase in ketones.

Myth #5: The Keto Diet Is the Most Effective Weight Loss Strategy

In case you hadn't heard, there isn't a "magic bullet" diet that works for everyone. Keto is not always the perfect diet for you just because your buddy lost weight on it, or it seems like everyone is talking about it. The most common misconception I see in my line of work these days is that the ketogenic diet is the holy grail of weight loss. The truth is that while it's tempting to try the latest fad diet, the key to long-term success is settling on a healthy eating pattern that you can stick to AND having an answer to two questions. What measures will I take to LOSE weight? What am I going to do to MAINTAIN the weight loss life-long? Those should be two different answers as you don't want to LIVE on a diet.

Fat Is Not the Enemy

Repeat after me "The only thing that is really bad for me is eating too much saturated fat and trans fat from processed foods." I know it's popular to hate fat and think that there are no healthy kinds, but this is very false! Take the creamy, deliciousness of avocado as an example. It is rich in beneficial fats that support our body's ability to absorb nutrients, produce hormones, protect organs, produce energy, develop cells, and insulate against cold. However, if you're not an avocado fan and aren't sure how to tell healthy fats from harmful ones, you're not alone in your bafflement.

Here, I've sifted through the nonsense to tell you which fats will help you achieve your objectives and which ones you should stay away from. Let's start off by discussing healthy fats. The body benefits particularly from the naturally occurring fats found in whole foods. Fats are the last to exit the digestive system, making them the most satisfying since they are both satiating and a source of energy. As a result, fats, particularly those made from real fats, can help us feel filled for longer and prevent us from overeating. What kinds of fats are thus worth watching out for? Well, to begin with, unsaturated fat is the nutritional facts' golden child.

In terms of health advantages, this kind of fat gets an A+. It falls into two groups: monounsaturated fats (MUFAs) and polyunsaturated fats (PUFAs). PUFAs have been shown to raise good cholesterol levels while simultaneously lowering LDL cholesterol levels (HDL). Plus, the risk of developing heart disease is decreased by the consumption of PUFAs. That is three big wins already! The omega-3 and omega-6 fatty acids that are good for the heart may be found in PUFAs. Hello, beautiful skin and lustrous hair, as well as a plethora of other health advantages! While keeping HDL levels the same, MUFAs may lower LDL. Moreover, several studies suggest they may lessen the dangers of cardiovascular disease. Over the years, you've probably heard that saturated fat raises Cholesterol levels, making it a bad food choice. However, recent research indicates that consuming more saturated fat is also linked to an increase in HDL, which lowers overall cholesterol levels.

At the moment, fewer than 10% of our daily calories should come from saturated fat, according to Health and Human Services (HHS) and the U.S. Department of Agriculture (USDA). Researchers, however, are advocating for revisions to this guideline since replacing our preferred lipids with processed carbohydrates may have unintended negative consequences. In fact, a meta-analysis led by (Dehghan et al., 2017) found that replacing saturated fat with refined carbohydrates like white rice and bread may raise the risk of cardiovascular disease. On the other hand, consuming more fat overall (both saturated and unsaturated) was linked to a reduced risk. The key is moderation; eating healthy doesn't require that you wrap every meal in bacon, but it also doesn't need you to avoid that whole-milk cappuccino. (You should cut down on the bread and butter and try to avoid eating too many refined carbohydrates and saturated fats at once.) What makes fat saturated? At room temperature, test the consistency. When left at room temperature, saturated fats remain solid whereas unsaturated fats remain liquid. Taking a look at the processing and packaging of the fat is a good way to get a sense of which fats are good for you. Bad fats are more likely to be present in prepackaged, processed meals. Good fats are more likely to be found in whole, unprocessed foods. Therefore, some saturated fats to consider eating are things like full-fat dairy products like butter, cheese, and cream, lard, and solid oils like palm, kernel, and coconut. True, our bodies need fat to function properly, but not all fats are the same. Fats are a great source of energy, and as long as we stay away from the unnatural trans fats found in fried meals and pastries, we should be good to go.

However, it's also OK and sometimes even advantageous to eat naturally occurring trans fats, such as those present in various meat and dairy products. Humans have been consuming these natural trans fats for ages after all, unlike synthetic trans fats. Therefore, as we've seen, fat can be a healthy element of your plan whether you're aiming to lose weight or maintain your present weight on the scale. However, this does not imply that you should rely only on fats for ALL of your nutritional needs. Because fat has a higher proportion of calories per gram than other macronutrients, eating too much of it may contribute to weight gain. Each gram of fat contains about 9 calories. The calorie content of both protein and carbohydrates is four. For the body to be well nourished, the diet must be balanced and include high-quality fats.

Fact 4:

Control Constipation—You Won't See This in the Books for Youngins

If you have ever suffered from constipation, you know how awful it can be. Constipation is one of the most frequent Gastrointestinal issues among US adults. Every year, at least 2.5 million individuals seek medical attention for constipation. Less than three bowel motions per week or stool movements that are difficult to pass are signs of constipation. This may lead to extra unnecessary time spent using the toilet and straining. Constipation is often seen as a symptom of an underlying illness, rather than a disease since its causes differ. Constipation may have many causes, but dehydration and a lack of fiber in the diet are the two common ones.

Constipation may also be brought on by stress, hormonal changes, spinal injuries, muscular issues, malignancies, and structural issues with the digestive system, among other, more severe conditions. The range of the total gut transit is about between 10 and 73 hours. However, the number of bowel movements you have in a given day is impacted by a variety of factors, including your age, gender, eating and exercise routines, as well as your current state of health. Although three or fewer times per week may be detrimental, there is no suggested minimum number of bowel movements. People over 50 and women are more likely to have constipation. This is especially true for the elderly, who, in comparison to their younger selves, are less likely to engage in physical activity, have slower metabolisms, and have weaker muscular contractions all throughout their digestive tract. The use of some drugs by older individuals, particularly when their health isn't being taken care of, tends to make them constipated. And when it comes to women, those who are pregnant are the ones who are most likely to be affected by it.

Pregnant women are more prone to constipation due to changes in their hormones. Because the growing baby puts pressure on the bowels, they move more slowly during pregnancy and sometimes even after. Not being able to poop doesn't mean you stop craving food, and this can easily result in weight gain. This uncomfortable feeling of not being able to poop when you really want leads many to turn to laxatives. People use laxatives, which are drugs, to assist in accelerating bowel movements or to loosen up a stool in order to make passing easier. Additionally, they are becoming a well-liked weight reduction technique. There is a widespread belief that using laxatives may facilitate an increased frequency of bowel movements, which in turn can make weight reduction more rapid, straightforward, and uncomplicated. And while laxatives have been shown to hasten weight reduction, this effect is only short-lived. Many different forms of laxatives achieve their desired effects by drawing water from the body into the intestines. This enables the stool to absorb more water and move more smoothly through the digestive tract. The only weight you will lose with this strategy is the water you pass via your bowels. The idea that laxatives are a useful tool for managing weight lacks any strong supporting data for long-term use. You don't necessarily need drugs to cure your constipation unless it's chronic, then in that case I would advise consulting your doctor. If not, though, there are still other better and healthier alternatives to treating constipation, which I go into depth about below.

Consider Magnesium Citrate

Magnesium Citrate is an all-natural supplement used to help bowel movements. It effectively binds the food in your gut to help carry it along the way at a reasonable rate. Typically, this is the job done by carbohydrates. If you are on a reduced carbohydrate diet, you may then need to supplement with Magnesium Citrate to temporarily take over this job. Brief bouts of constipation may be alleviated with the use of magnesium citrate. When you go to the bathroom more often, your stool gets softer and easier to pass. Magnesium citrate is a widely used, straightforward treatment for sporadic constipation when administered as directed. And for people with no health concerns, magnesium citrate is typically safe. Therefore, unless you consume too much of it, it shouldn't create urgency or sudden visits to the toilet. You don't need a prescription to get it, and you can find it at most stores like Walmart or Target although amazon has the best versions I have found.

Water, as noted in Fact number one, is very vital and possibly the greatest drink for helping with constipation relief. Drinking more water makes the most sense since chronic dehydration can lead to constipation. Water not only keeps you hydrated, but it also stimulates digestion. Some persons who suffer from chronic idiopathic constipation or indigestion (also known as dyspepsia) believe that sparkling water is even more beneficial than regular tap water in easing their symptoms. However, fizzy drinks like sugary soda should be avoided since they might have negative health impacts and may exacerbate constipation. Magnesium citrate in greater dosages is often prescribed by doctors as a colon cleanse prior to surgery. If someone consumes too much of the substance, it may have a strong impact. If you decide to use magnesium citrate, be sure to follow all dosing and storage directions provided by the manufacturer. Magnesium Citrate tablets are best with zero additives if possible. Avoid gel caps or liquids as they may have added unnecessary ingredients. Take it at bedtime.

Who Ought to Stay Away From Magnesium Citrate?

Most individuals can safely take magnesium citrate in the right amounts; however, there are certain people who should not. If you have a renal illness, nausea, stomach discomfort, vomiting, a sudden change in your bowel habits that has lasted more than a week, or if you are on a low-sodium or restricted-sodium diet, see your doctor before taking any magnesium citrate. Some drugs may be less effective when used with magnesium citrate because it might reduce their absorption. For instance, magnesium citrate may prevent some HIV medicines from functioning effectively if you are taking them. Therefore, find out from your doctor if any supplements or prescriptions you are taking might be affected by magnesium citrate. If you're experiencing rectal bleeding, then you shouldn't be using magnesium citrate. It should also be avoided by those who have had certain surgeries or have particular medical conditions. Magnesium citrate should not be used by anybody who often has prolonged bouts of constipation. Only mild or infrequent instances of constipation can be safely treated with magnesium. It is not meant for continued usage. The reason is that the body might develop a tolerance to magnesium citrate, making it difficult to defecate without the use of laxatives, if it is used on a frequent basis. To discover long-term treatments for their symptoms, anybody with persistent constipation should speak with their doctor.

Another Reason Why You Should Get All of Your Steps In

It's natural to want to curl up in the fetal position and hold your stomach when constipation strikes, but getting up off your bed and moving about will benefit you a great deal more. Physical exercise is perhaps one of the best lifestyle tricks for maintaining regularity and relaxing your bowels. It encourages the muscles in the gut wall to spontaneously contract by including frequent moderate-to-vigorous exercise in your daily routine. Jogging, water aerobics, and yoga are all examples of physical exercise, but even brisk walking can help with constipation difficulties. To successfully acquire fitness and good health, walk at a speed that is dictated by your metabolic rate. If you're told to walk at a brisk pace, all that implies is that you should walk a little quicker than usual. Your fitness level has a significant role in determining your pace. 100 steps per minute, or 3 to 3.5 miles per hour, is what most fitness professionals define as a brisk walking speed. Therefore, a great method to boost your physical activity is to go on brisk walks, which are considered moderate-intensity exercise. This kind of physical activity increases your heart rate, causes you to breathe more rapidly, and promotes good cardiovascular health. (Tantawy et al., 2017) examined middle-aged obese women who had persistent constipation for a period of 12 weeks. When compared to the control group that did not engage in any physical exercise, the first group's constipation symptoms and quality of life scores improved more after three weeks of walking on a treadmill for 60 minutes each time. Constipation is also related to an unbalanced gut bacterial population.

(Morita et al., 2019) conducted a research study in which they compared the makeup of gut microbes in the two groups to examine the impact of fast walking vs workouts that developed trunk muscles (such as planks). The research showed that aerobic exercises like brisk walking can increase the amount of Bacteroides in the gut, which are an important part of good gut bacteria. Studies have shown that people feel better when they walk quickly for at least 20 minutes every day, most days of the week. Recommendations for how long people should walk at a brisk pace differ.

What to do first

It's still crucial to consult your healthcare practitioner before beginning any walking program, even when walking may be exactly what you need at the moment. If you take any drugs or have any medical issues, then seeing a doctor is even more crucial. Some examples of this include experiencing lightheadedness, faintness, or difficulty breathing when on foot. If you take any drugs or have any medical issues, then seeing a doctor prior to beginning a vigorous exercise plan is recommended. To avoid hurting yourself, remember to never ignore your body's cues and do so much that you risk injury. To help you remain focused, look for a walking buddy who is also willing to serve as your accountability partner. Think about giving yourself non-food rewards when you achieve your objectives. This will make you feel proud, and you'll most likely want to continue. To track your daily speed and steps, you can use an app or a speedometer. Another option is to investigate if there are any walking groups in your area. Working out with other people is always more fun, plus you end up doing more workouts. Make the commitment to begin walking your way to improved health right now, no matter how you choose to go about it.

Why Leafy Green Vegetables Are Great

In some situations, the simplest of explanations will do the trick. Making a big salad with spinach and other leafy greens can help with constipation. This is because they hold a lot of insoluble fiber which has also been shown to reduce IBS symptoms. Insoluble fiber levels are often high in vegetables and certain fruits. Insoluble fiber doesn't break down in water or digestive fluids, so it mostly stays the same as it moves through the digestive system. Insoluble fiber is not a source of calories since it is not at all digested, but on the other hand, when soluble fiber reaches the stomach and intestines, it dissolves in water and digestive juices. The bacteria in the large intestine then break it down into a gel-like material, releasing gasses and a few calories in the process.

Consuming a lot of insoluble fiber while your stomach is inflamed is similar to rubbing a wire brush against an open cut, even though soluble fiber may be relaxing for the gut. That hurts, and it's not fun. If you like kale, arugula, and spinach in your salads rather than iceberg lettuce, give it a try. However, in addition to being high in fiber, green vegetables like spinach, broccoli, and Brussels sprouts are also excellent providers of vitamins C and K as well as folate. Stools made with these greens are heavier and have more mass, making it simpler for the intestines to move them along. Cooked spinach provides 4.7 grams of fiber, or 19% of the RDI, per cup (180 grams). If you want to increase the amount of spinach in your diet, you may make a pie, quiche, or soup using spinach as the main ingredient.

To increase the fiber content of salads or sandwiches, raw baby spinach or delicate greens may be used. Also, Brussels sprouts are very healthy. Just five sprouts give you 14% of your daily fiber needs and only 41 calories. They taste great hot or cold, and you can cook them by boiling, steaming, grilling, or roasting, and a single cup of broccoli has 2.4 grams of fiber (91 grams). This is 10%

of the recommended daily intake of fiber. It's versatile enough to be used in both hot and cold dishes, from salads to stews to raw additions to hot soups. Because it can't be digested, insoluble fiber helps prevent constipation by sticking to other parts of the digestive process that are getting ready to form stool and by soaking up liquids while it rests in the digestive system. Its presence speeds up the movement and digestion of waste, which lowers the risk of constipation and GI blockage.

Smooth Moves Tea

The natural laxative known as Smooth Move tea is a combination of organic herbs that is sold as a tea. It is supposed to help cure constipation in as little as six to twelve hours after taking it. The main ingredient is senna, a strong plant that grows in Africa and India. It is a well-liked component of constipation cure medicines due to its natural laxative effects. The active ingredient in senna, called sennoside, causes your bowels to contract and helps increase the amount of water and electrolytes in your colon, both of which help you go to the bathroom. Licorice, bitter fennel, cinnamon, ginger, coriander, and sweet orange are other components in Smooth Move tea. These herbs are designed to ease gastrointestinal discomfort and lessen cramping. Smooth Move tea preparation calls for 8 ounces (240 ml) of boiling water to be poured over a tea bag, followed by 10-15 minutes of steeping time with the lid on the mug. Teas that make you poop, like Smooth Move, are sometimes used to help people lose weight. This kind of tea causes bowel movements and hinders the body's ability to absorb water from your colon again. So, it may help you go to the bathroom and make you lose fluids, which can both help reduce bloating and give you a sense of lightness. Smooth Move tea's principal component is senna, a natural laxative that has been used for hundreds of years. It causes bowel movements to be more frequent, heavier, and softer. Smooth Move tea may also help keep you from getting hemorrhoids because it makes going to the bathroom easier.

Fact 5:

Everyone Exercise

We have already covered Macros and the importance of the right balance of certain foods and not just calories, now it's time to hit the other half of the equation- exercise. Food has approximately 70% of the power to help you lose weight and maintain it. The other 30% is moving! I'm sure just hearing the word "exercise" is bound to make some people uncomfortable. Everyone who's ever tried to look for ways to lose extra pounds, whether it be from a web search or by asking their doctor, has virtually been told the same thing, that dieting and exercise are your two best shots! It's not just an annoying cliche; it actually holds a lot of truth behind it that no one can really deny. If you want to lose weight or keep it off, then you need to make exercise a regular part of your life. When you try to lose weight, the more you exercise, the more calories your body "burns off" or uses for energy.

When you cut back on the number of calories you eat and increase the number of calories you burn through exercise, this is called a "calorie deficit." A lot of evidence suggests that regular physical exercise is one of the best methods for maintaining low body weight, if not the best. Being in a calorie deficit while eating the proper percentages and quantities of Macros along with moderate exercise is the key to lifelong weight loss and maintenance. Aerobic exercise, also known as cardio, is a favorite among those looking to trim down. Many people like activities like walking, jogging, cycling, and swimming, for example, because they get the job done. But compared to lifting weights, aerobic exercises don't do much for your muscle growth. It burns calories quite well, though. (Donnelly et al., 2013) performed a 10-month study that looked at how exercising without dieting affected 141 adults who were obese or overweight. The test subjects were split into three groups, and they were not told to eat less. 4.3% of the participants burned 400 calories in each cardio session (5 times per week), and 5.7% of the participants burned 600 calories in each session (5 times per week) reducing body weight, respectively.

The exercise-free control group really put on 0.5% of their body weight. Several studies have also shown that cardio is a good way to lose body fat, especially the dangerous belly fat that is linked to a higher risk of type 2 diabetes and heart disease. So, if you keep your macros in the appropriate ratio and quantity and add exercise to your life, it will really help you lose weight faster. It will improve your metabolic health as well. The best combination I have found to actually lose weight after 40 is to food cycle. Do a period of time where you are at a lower macro quantity and not doing much exercise. A 20-minute walk per day is perfect. Then go through a period of time where you are both the food and the exercise. Build those muscles! Food Cycling is a great way to beat plateaus.

What Exercise Routine Is Best for You

The Physical Activity Guidelines for Americans say that people should do at least 150 minutes per week of moderate aerobic activity, 75 minutes per week of vigorous aerobic activity, or an equal mix of the two. So, the goal is to be active for 30 minutes at a moderate level five days a week. But I don't advise setting that objective right away for the majority of people, especially those who are new to exercising. Instead, gradually increase your activity level to create a habit that you can maintain. Creating and maintaining an exercise program requires serious mental work. If you set too high a goal for how long you want to work out, it might be hard to stay motivated. Start by working out for shorter amounts of time, like 5 to 10 minutes, so that your body can get used to the idea of regular exercise. Also, even a short session of exercise can improve your sense of self-worth, lift your spirits, and give you a sense of accomplishment. So, my standard advice is to take baby steps.

The biggest problem is getting into the habit of working out regularly, and five minutes a day can help you do that. You'll be surprised at how much better you feel after you've gotten into this routine. Consistently following a program is key to making it successful and yielding benefits. Always remember that, especially on those days when you really don't want to work out, and trust me, there will be those days, but you can do it! It's a shame that so many people who are new to working out get discouraged because they think they need to start off strong. No, it is entirely OK to begin at your own speed and have shorter workout durations. If you're just getting into the habit of jogging, for instance, don't force yourself to jog for an hour on the first day! All this will do is make you too exhausted to go running the following day since your body, which isn't acclimated to this new way of life, will be in shock and need time to adjust. Keep in mind that gradual and long-lasting growth is best. But if you can make a commitment, I suggest starting with 20 minutes of exercise every day.

A stroll, a run, yoga, stretching, Pilates, core work, or HIIT workouts are all excellent forms of exercise to start with. If you begin with 20 minutes, you will have sufficient time to warm up, reach your peak performance, and then transition into the cool-down phase. At some point, spending up to 30 minutes a day at least on working out is preferable, but my adage is that progress comes slowly but surely. Choose an activity goal that you can handle and stick with it. Once you've been able to commit to 20 minutes of activity every day for a few weeks, I suggest you fine-tune your workout plan by focusing on your goals. Most of the time, my clients are under a lot of stress and have excess belly fat. As a result, I advise picking an activity that reduces tension. Going on a stroll, working out with HIIT, or having fun by dancing while you exercise are all great options.

To Muscle up or Not to Muscle Up?

In a well-balanced recomposition of the body, losing weight and gaining muscle go hand in hand. When you lose weight and fat, especially in your stomach, your metabolism speeds up. This gives you the energy to train harder and build nice, lean muscles. Muscle, being the highly metabolically active tissue that it is, also helps with fat reduction. This is because our basal metabolic rate (BMR), or the number of calories your body burns at rest, increases as we gain muscle. So simply, the more muscle you have, the more fat you stand to lose. As I mentioned above, food cycling helps if you are both looking to lose weight and build muscle.

If you lose weight (also known as fat), you'll not only start to notice results sooner, but you'll also benefit from things like better sleep and a better mood. Although if you choose to prioritize muscle growth first, don't be surprised if you gain some weight in the early stages. In fact, you can count on this happening, but it shouldn't be a cause for concern. It's just that your muscle fibers are under stress from a new training routine. This results in some inflammation and tiny micro rips, commonly known as "microtrauma." This initial weight gain is what discourages a lot of women and may even lead some to give up on their good diet and exercise routines entirely. When you reduce your body fat percentage, you make your body's hormones more stable, which paves the way for improved insulin sensitivity and enhanced muscle-building potential (the way your body responds to and processes blood sugar).

When your primary goal is to build muscle mass, this will speed up your metabolism and make it easier to lose weight. Both are great goals. Strength training and eating more protein may help you keep as much muscle as possible while you lose fat and change the shape of your body by going after fat stores first. For long-term weight loss and fitness success, it's important to focus on both lowering body fat and building lean muscle mass. If you have a well-rounded plan for your workouts and food, you can reach both of your goals at the same time. But ultimately, your body fat percentage will determine this. So, if you're overweight or obese, which is defined as a body fat percentage of over 25% for men and over 32% for women, you should aim for weight loss first. And besides, it's way more difficult to try to grow muscle while also trying to cut body fat if you already have a lot of it. Your body will be more receptive to gaining muscle initially if you have a lower body fat percentage because you don't need to remove as much fat. You already know that losing weight has many advantages, including better sleep, lower blood pressure, lower risk of heart disease and diabetes, reduced blood sugar and cholesterol levels, and so forth. However, losing weight can also give you more energy and make you feel better about yourself overall. There will be less wear and tear on your ligaments and cartilage if you maintain a healthy body weight, which will make it easier to train hard and gain muscle.

The process of gaining muscle is often slower than the process of losing fat, which means that you will notice the effects of fat reduction much more quickly. If you focus on reducing your body fat first, you will be able to see your underlying muscle structure more clearly, which will make it easier for you to sculpt and define your physique. While it's true that building muscle may help you burn more calories because of the metabolic boost that comes with it, doing so takes time and a lot of work. Putting on muscle already takes women longer than males, so I would recommend shedding the pounds first before beginning to sculpt your beautiful physique. Gaining muscle mass increases your resting metabolic rate, which may be a significant help in the fight against obesity since it accounts for anywhere from 60-75% of our daily caloric expenditure. Putting forth the effort to eat a high-protein diet and work out in order to gain muscle mass is a double win for your waistline.

For instance, a study by (Longland et al., 2016) looked at individuals who consistently worked out hard and were in a caloric deficit. The study eventually concluded that those who consumed more protein lost 27% more fat and gained eight times as much lean muscle mass. Building muscle has many advantages beyond just boosting metabolism, though, including bettering your cardiovascular and joint health, lowering your risk of diabetes and certain cancers, enhancing your mental well-being, and enhancing bone health and strength, which reduces your risk of osteoporosis and falls. Whether you prioritize fat loss or muscle building depends on your unique health status and desired outcomes from your exercise program. To guarantee you're losing mostly fat and not hard-earned muscle, though, make sure your diet contains at least 0.7 grams of protein per pound of body weight (or 1.6 grams per kilogram). It's probably also a good idea to get someone like your accountability buddy to, well, keep you accountable. For best results, include enjoyable activities in your life. Ideally, this would include a mix of aerobic exercises, such as a HIIT workout, an interval workout, a long walk, or a run, as well as 2-3 days of strength training per week to maintain muscle mass. Strength training with heavier weights and fewer repetitions strengthens muscles, while aerobic endurance workouts like jogging, cycling, or brisk walking uphill improve stamina and allow you to train more often witho out. To promote muscle building, be sure to eat enough high-quality proteins throughout the day, with at least 20 grams of protein at each meal, such as fish, chicken, turkey, beans, lentils, and tofu. For the absolute best in a personalized macro and fitness program, you may reach me at www.lifelongmetaboliccenter.com.

Fact 6:

Habits to Hijack

There is no denying that humans are creatures of habit. We love following the same routine over and over again. For instance, most of us buy the same food every day from our "usual" supermarket and probably even cook the same meals, but if you want to become healthy and drop those pounds, you'll have to switch things up, abandon some of your unhealthy old routines, and adopt some new ways of thinking. The only issue is that we have a really hard time breaking old habits once we get used to them. People usually don't want to make positive changes to their diets because they are used to the foods and drinks they already eat and drink and are afraid of what might happen if they make these changes. Old habits are difficult to break, even when you know they're bad for you.

A habit is a learned behavior that develops through time and is stronger than a newer habit you are attempting to adopt." Even the most disciplined eaters can revert to old habits when under duress. When someone feels helpless or vulnerable, their instincts often take over, even if they want to do the right thing. Things may be going well until you reach a hard patch and are overcome by boredom, loneliness, sadness, or tension, which will have you reaching for those honey buns. Being self-aware is the first step to changing unhealthy eating and exercise habits. The second step is to figure out why these habits started in the first place. The third step is to make a plan for making the necessary changes over time. By breaking the process into smaller pieces, you can make it easier to change your behavior in a way that will last. If you can make little changes over time, you'll soon be on the path to a healthier diet and a trimmer body. Changing to a healthy diet might be scary at first. However, success is more likely after you experience the positive effects of eating healthily and realize how delicious and nutritious food can be. If you stick with it, your taste for unhealthy foods will shift and eventually disappear.

Some habits I have taught my patients to ditch are stress eating through habit replacement, caving to cravings, and allowing yourself to keep your excuses. We covered habit replacement already. That's a MAJOR one. Cravings can be real or fake. Real cravings are when your body is sending you signals there is a need. One very common one is water. Another is fat. Fat makes you feel full, so if you have tried water, have a little healthy fat and see if it kicks that craving. Fake cravings may just be boredom or thinking about food. Change your mind and stomp those fake cravings. By disallowing your excuses, you can totally change your habits. Become a solution-finder rather than an excuse-maker. Every problem has a solution. Set your mind right and your body is soon to follow. If you find yourself unable to do this alone, there are amazing mental health professionals out there who are trained at retraining the brain. Reach out!

How To Change Your Habits

As the rock of life rolls along, we have gathered the "moss" of some bad habits. It's not too late to dump those and adopt new good habits. It takes three stages.

- Reminder (the trigger that triggers the action) This might be a deliberate action, like flushing the toilet, or a mood, like anxiety.
- Routine (the behavior itself that is related to the trigger; the action you execute): For example, flushing the toilet prompts you to wash your hands, while being anxious prompts you to bite your fingernails. Routine behavior may develop through repeated actions.
- Reward is the advantage gained from carrying out the activity (the benefit gained from carrying out the behavior). When there is a reward for an action, it becomes ingrained.

The "3 R's of Habit Change" concept has been repeatedly demonstrated by behavioral psychology experts. BJ Fogg, a Stanford professor, was the first to introduce me to the concept of habit formation. I learned about it in the latest edition of *The Power of Habit by Charles Duhigg*. The three phases of the "Habit Loop" are referred to as cue (reward), routine, and reward in Duhigg's book *How Habits Work* (Charles Duhigg, 2017). He says that almost any behavior can be changed with his techniques, though it might take some time and work. The structure is as follows: 1) figure out the routine (what needs to change), 2) try out different rewards, 3) find the cue, and 4) come up with a plan.

First, You Need to Pinpoint the Routine

In order to break a bad habit, you must first identify the feedback loop that keeps you engaging in it and then actively seek alternatives. Consider the following scenario: Say you've just clocked off from work, and you and your colleagues decide to go to a cafe to hang out and relax from the work day. This isn't anything new for you guys; in fact, you guys come to this particular cafe almost every day after work to enjoy some food, chat and laugh. All seems well and good until you realize that every time you're at this cafe, you have the nasty habit of purchasing a slice of their specially-made cheesecake (sometimes even more). Now, suppose you've put on some weight as a result of this routine. In fact, imagine this habit has led to an exact 11-pound weight increase. You have made several attempts to break this habit, even going so far as to write the words "no more cheesecake" on a post-it note that you pasted on your desk in an attempt to motivate yourself to quit. You see that letter every day before you leave the office, yet you still manage to accept your coworker's invitation, drive to the cafe, purchase that cheesecake, and indulge in it all the while conversing with coworkers at the seating section.

At first you feel great, you and your colleagues are sharing stories, enjoying good food, and just having a relaxing time overall after the work day. But after an hour when you all decide to go home, you start to feel guilty, and that good feeling turns into a regretful one. You feel great for a little while because of the dopamine receptors in your brain, but that all comes crashing down soon, and you end up feeling guilty. You make a commitment to yourself that you will have the willpower to resist tomorrow. It will be different tomorrow, but it never is, and the habit returns the next day. In order to begin correcting this habit, how do you identify it first? by identifying the habit loop of course. The first order of business is to recognize the pattern. The most obvious part of this cheesecake situation is the routine since it is the behavior you want to change.

Every day around five o'clock, you get up from your desk, make plans with your coworkers to meet up at the local cafe, where you enjoy a slice of cake while also having long and fun conversations with your work friends, and then repeat the next day. Thus, this is what you include in the loop. Following that, ask yourself several questions that may not be immediately apparent: What signals the start of this routine? Is it a drop in blood sugar? Boredom? Hunger? The cake itself? a shift in scenery? Stress from work? Stress at home? getting to know your coworkers? Or maybe that sugar rush that gives you a surge of energy? what is the prize? To find the answer, some trial and error will be required.

Experiment With Rewards in Step Two

The effectiveness of rewards lies in their ability to quell desires. However, we often aren't aware of the desires that motivate our actions. Most desires seem obvious when we look back on them, but it is very hard to tell when they are in charge of us. It helps to try out different rewards to figure out which cravings are behind certain behaviors. It's possible that this will take several days, up to a week, or even longer. During that time, you shouldn't put any pressure on yourself to make a significant adjustment; instead, you should see yourself as a researcher who is in the process of gathering information. When you sense the need to go to the cafe and purchase a cheesecake or any other dessert on the first day of your trial, change your routine so that it produces a new reward. For example, when you're at the cafe, instead of buying cheesecake, you could buy a coffee or a piece of fruit, eat it, then converse with friends before going home. Remember not to buy anything else but these two items. The next day, avoid going to the cafe altogether and instead go for an after-work jog or run with music. The next day, get your usual cheesecake. Then, as the next day rolls around, try something new, like a salad. Then the next day, instead of going to the cafe, you could invite a couple of your work friends somewhere else where there is no food that can tempt you. You get the gist.

It doesn't matter what you decide to do in place of purchasing that cake. Testing several theories can help you identify which desire is responsible for your pattern. Do you yearn for the desert itself? Are you just exhausted from work and need to unwind a little bit before going home? If so, go for a walk rather than giving in to the need to eat. Is the cake only a pretext for you to visit the cafe and mingle with your work friends? Did the workday tire you out and now you're in need of some energy in the form of sugar? (If yes, coffee or tea should be a better option.) Or are you really just hungry (in which case a salad or banana might also satisfy your hunger)? You may employ a tried-and-true method to search for trends as you try four or five different rewards: When you return home after each practice, write down on a piece of paper the first three ideas that spring to mind. They might be feelings, unrelated ideas, observations about how you're feeling, or even simply the first three words that come to mind. Next, set a 15-minute alarm on your computer or watch. When it sounds, ask yourself if you still want that piece of cake. Even if the three items are just words, it's still vital to record them for two reasons. It first compels you to briefly become aware of your thoughts and feelings.

Writing three words forces you to pay attention for a moment, just like how Mandy, the nail-biter in fact 3, carried around a note card with hash marks on it to make her aware of her repeated cravings. Additionally, studies demonstrate that jotting down a few words makes it easier to remember what you were thinking at the time in the future. It's particularly intriguing that taking notes seems to make crucial information easier for us to recall, and that the better our notes are, the more likely we are to do so. When you reread your notes at the conclusion of the experiment, your scrawled words will automatically produce a wave of remembering, and it will be much simpler to recall what you were thinking and experiencing at that precise time. And if you're wondering about the 15-minute alarm, it's because the goal of these tests is to identify the reward that you really want. If you still want the cake after chatting with coworkers, then your behavior probably isn't motivated by a need for human interaction. And if you still have the urge to go walk around while listening to music after eating your cheesecake, then your behavior isn't likely to be motivated by a sugar craving. But do notice if you really want to go get another slice of cake after those 15 minutes, because that's a sign of a sugar craving. But if you're happy with the end of your day after spending time with friends, even if you didn't have your piece of cake that night, that means you've found that "social engagement" is what your habit was looking for as a reward. Perhaps it was boredom and a need for a change of scenery that caused you to want human interaction, and that kind of socializing obviously centers around eating and chatting. So it's really easy to get sidetracked when in a conversation like this. But the good news is, you've identified the reward! To change a habit, you need to figure out what you really want, which you can do by practicing with different rewards. Knowing the pattern and the reward isn't enough to break the cycle; you also need to find out the cue, or "what is triggering you?"

Isolate the Cue in Step Three

A University of Western Ontario psychologist sought to solve a topic that has puzzled social scientists for years: why do some eyewitnesses of crimes misremember what they see? It goes without saying that eyewitness accounts are crucial. Despite this, research shows that eyewitnesses' memories are typically inaccurate. They claim that the killer had black hair and green eyes while, for example, he really had blonde hair and blue eyes. Others, however, have a near-perfect recollection of atrocities they saw as an eyewitness.

Researchers proposed two theories as to why some remember and others don't: either some individuals just have superior recollections, or crimes that take place in well-known settings are simpler to remember. However, such hypotheses were disproven because those with good and bad memory, or who were more or less acquainted with the scene of a crime, were equally likely to recall anything incorrectly. A distinct strategy was used by the University of Western Ontario psychologist (Will, 2022). By concentrating on what interrogators and witnesses had said rather than how they were saying it, she questioned if academics were doing it wrong. She had a sneaking suspicion that there were subliminal indications dictating how the questions were asked. She searched through recordings and videotapes of witness interviews for these indicators, but she was unable to find any. She was unable to identify any trends since each interview was so chaotic due to the variety of facial expressions, questions asked, and emotions shown. So she had an idea: She produced a list of a few aspects she would pay attention to, including the tone of the questioner, the witness's facial expressions, and the distance between the witness and the questioner. She then deleted any material that would have drawn her attention away from those components. She reduced the television's volume so that she could only make out the tone of the questioner's voice rather than any spoken words. She covered the questioner's face with tape so that she could only see the witnesses' facial reactions. She measured their separation from one another by holding a tape measure up to the screen. And as soon as she began examining these particular components, patterns were obvious. She observed that officers often questioned witnesses who misremembered details in a kind, pleasant manner. The likelihood of misremembering increased when witnesses smiled more or sat closer to the person asking the questions. That is to say, eyewitnesses were more prone to distort the events that transpired when social indicators say "we are friends" (e.g., a soft tone, a kind expression). Maybe it was because such social signals made you want to satisfy the interrogator more than usual. However, what makes this experiment so significant is that hundreds of other researchers had already seen identical videos.

Although many intelligent individuals had seen the same correlations, no one had previously identified them. The reason was, each cassette had too much data to pick up on a slight hint. Except as soon as the psychologist made the decision to ignore all but three types of behavior and discard irrelevant data, the patterns were obvious. In many ways, our lives are identical. There is too much information coming at us as our behaviors develop, which is why it is so difficult to pinpoint the indicators that set off our habits. Is it hunger that drives you to have breakfast every morning at the same time? Or is it because it's 7:30? Or maybe it's because your kids are now eating? Or maybe you find that after you've gotten dressed, you have a greater tendency to eat breakfast. What motivates you to travel the same route to school every day even when you could go a different way? Is it the quickest path since there are the fewest roadblocks? or maybe it's all of the aforementioned? You're driving your child to school, but for some reason, you find yourself on the way to the office instead of the school's location. What was the trigger that made the habit of "driving to work" take hold instead of the habit of "driving to school"?

We may use the same method as the psychologist to pick out a signal from the background chatter by preparing ourselves to look for patterns in certain types of behavior. Fortunately, science may be of some assistance here. A majority of habitual cues, according to experiments, fall into one of five categories: location, time, other people, emotional state, and the action that comes right after it.

In order to identify the trigger for the habit of "going to the café and purchasing a cheesecake," you should note the following five factors as soon as the temptation strikes:

Where are you right now? (At the dining room table.) What is the time? (5:23 pm.) How do you feel at the moment? (happy that game night is taking place at the café.) Who else is in the area? (Katy, Ryan, Susie, and Michael.) What behavior came before the urge? (I wanted a cheesecake after seeing Susie enjoy one.)

Following day:

Where are you right now? (returning from my vehicle on foot.) What is the time? (5:18 pm.) How do you feel at the moment? (cheerful.) Who else is with you? (Michelle from accounting.) What behavior came before the urge? (Discuss office drama.)

Three days later:

Where are you right now? (Pier for businesses.) When is the time? (5:07 pm.) How are you feeling right now? (Excited to go unwind at the cafe despite being tired.) Who else is with you? (A few of my department's coworkers.) What behavior came before the urge? (The rest of the group is enthused.)

By day three, it ought to be obvious which cue sets off your habits. It was obvious which cue was setting off her cheesecake habit in the previous cheesecake example.

She wanted social interaction and the rest of the day off from work as her reward. According to the day's example above, the habit trigger occurred between 5:00 and 6:00

Step 4: Create a plan.

You can start to change the behavior after you've recognized your habit loop, which includes the reward motivating your activity, the signal causing it, and the pattern itself. By anticipating the cue and adopting an action that will result in the desired reward, you may switch to a better pattern. You should make a plan. We discovered that habits are decisions that we make consciously at one time but then automatically repeat, usually on a daily basis. So basically, a habit is an instinctive pattern that our brain follows, such as when we perceive a cue, we will do a routine in order to get a reward. We need to start making decisions once again in order to re-engineer that formula. And several studies have shown that having a strategy is the simplest approach to do this. In psychology, these tactics are known as "implementation intentions." Consider the habit of eating cheesecake in the early evening. We were able to determine that the cue in that instance was about 5:30 in the afternoon by using this framework. The routine was to stroll down to the parking lot with the employees, drive to the café, get a cheesecake, take a seat, and talk with a friend for at least an hour. Through trial and error, we discovered (as she did) that what she truly craved was the chance to spend time with her friends and connect without having to worry about anything else for at least a little while, and that cheesecake was just an excuse.

I suppose you might argue that the benefit was a brief escape. Therefore, you need to record a strategy in your diary along these lines: If my friends suggest going to the café at around 5:00 p.m., I'll decline the offer and instead ask them if they want to go on a leisurely trek with me. Set an alarm for a few minutes before 5:00 to ensure that you remember to do this. This will allow you to leave and avoid walking to the parking lot with them if accepting their offer proves to be too alluring. If you have the choice, you might also park your vehicle on the other side of the parking lot to avoid encountering them before leaving to go home. Even if this may not work right away, continue with your strategy. There may be times (particularly early on) when your discipline still needs work, and you could stray from the path, but those are the times when you must keep your eyes on your goal and persevere! You'll discover that the end of the tunnel is not completely dark and that cheesecake has nothing on you. It goes without saying, however, that certain habits might be harder to break than others. But we can start with this foundation. Change might take a very long time. Repeated failures and experimentation are sometimes necessary. But you can control a habit once you know how it works—after you identify the signal, the pattern, and the reward.

Emotional Eaters

People who eat due to emotional ups or downs are what we call "emotional eaters." Is emotional eating something you struggle with? Do you ever find yourself reaching for, or desiring, a specific meal when you're upset, unhappy, bored, or lonely? As an example, after a long day of stress, an emotional eater may have a strong need for chocolate. And to be completely honest, I think it's safe to say that all of us are sometimes guilty of "eating our emotions." When feelings become overwhelming, it's not uncommon for people to seek solace in food. It's only human to look for stress relief methods after all. And since we depend on food for survival, eating is naturally gratifying. The problem is that relying on food as a form of stress relief or emotional support isn't exactly beneficial to one's physical or mental well-being. Naturally, your physical state will be impacted by your emotional eating habits. In addition to the obvious effects of gaining weight, overeating can also sap your vitality, trigger headaches, and otherwise make you feel awful. The other problem is that eating isn't effective as a means of dealing with negative feelings. While there is no shortage of advice on how to deal with emotional eating, it's important to note that severe dietary regimens don't suit everyone. Many of us continue to struggle with emotional eating even after we have learned and committed certain dietary rules to memory, such as restricting ourselves to one meal a day or not eating after 6 p.m. For sure, such was the situation with my pal Jessica. She is one of the funniest and most hardworking people I know. After all, being one of the best attorneys in her legal firm requires some effort.

This firm handles a lot of important cases for some of the most powerful people in the country, so Jessica is under a lot of pressure at work. It's not unusual for her to spend many nights working and fretting about work, and regrettably, the way she copes with this stress is to eat all of the pastries in the fridge. She confided in me that the only things that make her feel better whenever she is feeling stressed at work are sweets of any kind (ice cream, cupcakes, cinnamon buns, etc.). Of course, every time she finished a bar of chocolate, for instance, she would quickly feel the need for another item, and this would simply keep happening. "I'm not sure what's wrong with me. I know I should stop, but at those times, it's as if sweets are the only thing that can distract me from overthinking. "I feel like a failure," she said. I told her not to be so harsh on herself and explained that when you need food and then satisfy that craving, you receive an internal injection of Dopamine—a feel-good hormone. And that she ate a cookie every time she felt that unpleasant feeling—stress. Your brain's reward system is active, and you are content. However, this only lasts for a short time, and when you come down from that transient high and realize you're still agitated, you'll automatically grab for another cookie, and so the cycle repeats. Even if the goal of food rules is to promote self-control, it's not unexpected that they don't always end up being effective in the case of emotional eating. If you're an emotional eater like Jessica, you may think you have no control over what and how much you eat. In most cases, a person's emotional eating has nothing to do with a lack of willpower. In actuality, you most likely have lots of it! When it comes to eating out of emotional distress, it's rarely the act of eating itself that's the issue. Don't forget that humans are natural eaters! It's human nature to want something comforting to eat! Actually, the problem isn't with your eating habits per se, but with the unpleasant emotion that drives you to use food as a consolation. You're less likely to be able to stop emotional eating until you deal with the feeling that's driving you to eat in a way that is constructive and really helps you deal with the feeling.

To Help You Kick Emotional Eating:

1. Identify the Conduct

    Recognizing that you are engaging in emotional eating is the first step in overcoming this problem. Learn to identify and accept emotional overeating for what it is so you may stop using food as a coping mechanism for emotions and start eating to satiate genuine hunger. What circumstances, locations, or emotions cause you to turn to food for comfort? Although it may sometimes be brought on by nice sensations, like rewarding oneself for reaching a goal or enjoying a special occasion, emotional eating is often associated with negative feelings. By realizing that the only reason you're eating right now is because you're feeling bad, you've already taken the first step toward getting rid of it. If you take the time to put your feelings into words on paper, you will have taken an even more significant step forward. This procedure may seem simple, even elementary. But in order to succeed in the long run, you must accept your conduct without criticizing yourself. The time has come to work very hard now. Here, judgment is not helpful to us. This just serves to exacerbate the problem. When you judge yourself harshly, you also experience intense feelings of shame and guilt, which only serve to increase your emotional burden and make it more difficult to work through your feelings. When you realize and accept that you are emotionally eating, remind yourself that you are a person who is feeling normal human emotions.

2. Find a way to deal with your emotional issue emotionally

When you want to stop stress eating or emotional eating, it helps to let yourself experience the emotion and then figure out a healthy way to deal with it. Like the example, we used above with the 3 R's. Now that you know what makes you turn to food when you're feeling down, you can go on to Step 2 and find a healthier way to deal with your emotions. Finding a more effective technique to deal with your feelings is the aim. Which begs the question: What is the best way to deal with your feelings? Well, this is a question that can only be answered on a case-by-case basis; here are some general suggestions for dealing with a range of typical emotions.

- Boredom: Try doing something different, like wrapping up an unfinished task, cleaning your house, or even just watching a movie or reading a book.

- Stress: breathing exercises, meditation, taking a quiet stroll, listening to calming music, and drinking water are all effective relaxation techniques.

- Anxiety: It might help to talk to a trusted friend, take a relaxing bath, play with your pet(s), or even see a professional. Even though it's true that some foods can help lower anxiety, it's best for people who have a problem with overeating to incorporate them into their diet rather than eat them on the spur of the moment because binge eating can actually make anxiety much worse from the food itself.

- Loneliness: Connect with friends or family by text, phone, or video chat.

- Sadness: try making a list of everything you're thankful for or watch a funny movie.

Trying to control your munching in the here and now is vital, but figuring out what's causing your stress in the first place is more crucial in the long run. Healthy routines like exercise, rest, and a balanced diet all serve as effective stress relievers.

3. Distinguish Between Emotional and Hunger Cues

It's not always easy to tell the difference between eating because you're hungry and emotional eating. By eating consciously and paying attention to hunger cues, you may learn to distinguish between the two and control your eating. But, to put it simply, physical hunger builds up slowly and correlates with the time since your last meal. while factors like stress, anxiety, or weariness cause emotional hunger. Emotional hunger is often your body's way of letting you know that you need solace or something calming. Assessing your level of hunger on a scale of one to 10 is a good practice exercise. You may rank your level of hunger as anything between one and four if you're not really hungry, or just slightly so. Before eating, wait until you are actually hungry at five (but don't let yourself get extremely hungry to the point of overeating).

4. Establish a Schedule

   Consistently adhering to a schedule of regularly spaced meals and, for some individuals, regularly spaced snacks, may help curb binge eating. Contrarily, erratic eating patterns are often problematic since they lead to impulsive and excessive eating. Some individuals plan their day around three main meals and two smaller meals, or "mini meals," spaced evenly throughout the day. The feeling of true hunger often sets in approximately three hours after the last meal. A little snack may be adequate at that point, depending on your eating habits and the time of day; if not, it's time for your next meal.

5. Replace With Healthy Behaviors

   If you're used to eating in response to emotional situations, make a list of new habits to replace eating as a response to stress. They should take about 2-5 minutes, about the same amount of time as eating a snack. Some examples may be:

soaking your feet in warm baking soda water, cleaning out a cabinet or closet, painting your nails, reading five pages in a book, etc. Do these, and you get the same dopamine "high" and a healthier outcome. When you retrain the habit of "stress eating" now, it will make keeping weight off later much easier. Walking is another easy, quick, and healthy substitute for emotional eating. You can walk normally, quickly, on a treadmill, or with your dog. Practicing a craft like knitting or felting not only provides a welcome diversion, they also provide an outlet for one's imagination and a means of making useful objects.

6. Examine Your Eating Habits

What you eat may not always matter as much as how you eat. More factors than just the particular items you choose to consume might contribute to emotional overeating, including overall food intake, attitude toward food, meal and snack balance, and individual eating patterns. Take stock of your eating habits, educate yourself on the differences between regular eating and emotional overeating, and come up with some new methods of self-help to deal with your mental and physical connections to food. It's important to practice saying "no" in order to succeed in forming healthier eating habits. This includes saying "no" to harmful meals as well as emotionally charged circumstances.

7. Change Your Eating Habits

Some individuals gain weight because they have unhealthy eating habits like skipping breakfast or eating late at night. But that doesn't mean you have to force yourself to have breakfast every morning, or that you can't eat anything at night if you really want to. But if your usual eating schedule isn't allowing you to slim down or keep your portions in check, you may want to try something different. Eating your major meal earlier in the day (for lunch) rather than later in the day (what may be considered conventional dinnertime) has been shown to aid with weight reduction and management in short-term trials. In other words, dine like a king (or queen) in the morning, and a princess (or beggar) in the afternoon.

8. Strike a Balance

In order to say that your life is well-balanced, you must be happy with all or almost all of its components. It implies that your physiological, psychological, and spiritual needs are being satisfied. A diet that is out of balance means that it either includes too few of the healthiest foods or too many of the unhealthiest ones. Emotional eating may also be a symptom of a deeper problem, such as a lack of self-care that manifests physically as illness, fatigue, or excess weight. Try to make changes in the parts of your life where you feel the most discontent in order to achieve a sense of equilibrium. Write these down. Score each section of your life and work on those with the lowest score first. This can help you keep from feeling overwhelmed and help to focus on one area at a time productively.

9. Collect Your Forces

Having a support system of loved ones and, if required, a therapist or coach may be just as crucial to your progress as your own drive and determination. Supporters can assist by encouraging you, suggesting better meal options, understanding the emotional roots of your overeating problems, and even assisting to defuse some of the emotional circumstances that cause your overeating. Create a support system of individuals who can listen, who can motivate, and inspire you, and who may even be willing to join you in your efforts to improve your health and wellness by cooking, walking, or working out. Social functions can make it difficult to stick to a diet, and if your life is rich in social outings, you will need a solution. Especially if someone in your life is a food pusher. Moms and grandmas are good at this. They often express love through food. In older generations, this may stem from a period in their own lives where food was scarce, so they don't want you to experience the same lack. Keep this in mind when responding. Enlist the help of someone else who will be with you at these functions. Kindly refuse and stick to your plan. It doesn't have to be dramatic or rude, but you will have to face it, so, this situation doesn't sabotage your progress.

10. Focus Inwards

You must always remind yourself that you are capable of completing any task at hand if you want to be successful. It's impossible to feel content and successful all the time; that's just not how life works. For instance, if you indulge in an emotional eating session, be kind to yourself and start again the next day. Make an effort to reflect on what went wrong and figure out what you can do to avoid this happening again. When you run into trouble, don't give up; instead, force yourself to keep looking for a way to solve the problem. Give yourself credit for the healthy lifestyle adjustments you've made, and keep your mind on the benefits of your new eating habits. While others may be of great assistance, it is up to you to identify your own abilities and utilize them to carry out the inner work and emotional work that you alone are capable of carrying out.

Fact 7:

Hunger Hacks

It's much easier said than done to eat healthily in order to lose weight. And if you've been trying to stick to a strict diet, you know how tempting it may be to revert to old eating habits. Some patients don't like keeping a food diary or skipping nightly ice cream while others don't see time in their schedule to exercise. One common issue is the feeling of hunger; not emotional eating, but truly feeling hunger. What, then, are some methods for regulating appetite and warding off unwelcome food cravings? It's crucial to keep in mind that using diet pills, herbal supplements, or crash diets to reduce weight might have detrimental long-term effects on your health. There are several natural methods you can use to help manage your hunger, but the first thing to do is determine if you are really, genuinely hungry in the first place.

How to Recognize When You're Really Hungry

Being "hungry" and "wanting something to eat" is not the same thing. You can tell the difference between real hunger and hunger caused by stress or emotions by a few clear signs. Start by answering the following questions: Is your tummy growling? Are you experiencing any "brain fog" or irritability? Have you seen a decrease in your energy levels? If you answered yes to any of these questions, you're probably experiencing real hunger. True hunger often manifests in these ways. In this state, your body is more likely to react positively to food, and you may experience an improvement in your mood after eating. Food, however, probably won't help you feel any less bored, angry, or sad if you're eating for reasons other than real hunger. And if it happens, you most likely won't experience that feeling for very long.

Best Techniques for Controlling Your Appetite

- *Get a lot of protein.* Consuming protein with each meal is a wonderful strategy to curb hunger pangs and eat less overall. In fact, among the three macronutrients (fats, carbohydrates, and protein), protein has been shown in several studies to have the greatest satiety-inducing effect. I always thought it was fat that was most satisfying and had read several studies stating that as well, so alas, we are back to getting a good balance of all three for the best results. These new studies say the hormone that causes hunger, ghrelin, is decreased by protein. Peptide YY, a hormone that makes you feel full, is also increased by it. These impacts on hunger may be quite potent. According to research that was conducted by (Weigle, 2022), increasing the amount of protein consumed from 15% to 30% of total calories caused overweight women to consume 441 fewer calories on a daily basis, even though they did not consciously limit anything. Foods that are high in protein are also low in calories per gram. Cutting down on carbs and fats may help you lose weight more quickly than cutting back on protein. It could be as easy as cutting down on the number of potatoes or grains you eat and adding a few more bites of fish or steak. You may also add foods like salmon, lean chicken, turkey, lentils, eggs, cottage cheese, Greek yogurt, and soybeans as high-protein meals.

- *Sip some coffee.* Both green tea and coffee have been shown to reduce hunger pangs and speed up the metabolic rate. But if you reach for these beverages, avoid those with excessive amounts of milk and/or sugar.

Some studies have shown that drinking coffee may help you eat less by reducing your hunger, delaying your stomach from emptying as quickly, and even influencing the hormones responsible for hunger. Plus, caffeine has been shown to promote fat-burning and support weight reduction. When caffeine is ingested, it increases the body's metabolism, thus temporarily reducing appetite. Thermogenesis, or the body's creation of heat and energy from the digestive processes, will be induced by caffeine. This means that for a short period of time, you will burn more calories because coffee encourages a stronger metabolic response from your body. In addition, compared to those who don't drink coffee, coffee drinkers may also be less prone to overeating during their next meal and throughout the day. It gives you something to sip on which fills your stomach and keeps your hands busy- also warm on cold winter days.

Eat plenty of high-fiber, water-rich meals to fill up. There are no calories in water or fiber. High-water-content meals with plenty of fiber are "bulky" and make you feel full because they take up more room in your stomach. Also, due to their high water and fiber content, the majority of vegetables—aside from those that are starchy like potatoes, corn, and peas—have relatively few calories per serving. You can also feel full at a relatively cheap calorie cost by eating watery fruits like melons and pineapple as well as rich fiber foods like berries.

Eat a lot of nuts. Protein, unsaturated fat, vitamin E, magnesium, and antioxidants are all abundant in nuts. If you're feeling hungry, grab a handful, and you'll soon forget you were hungry. Beware though of the serving size of nuts. They, along with nut butters are easy to overeat. By purchasing single-serving packets, you can eliminate overeating. Another tip is to get whatever serving size you intend to eat, close the container, and walk away before you start eating.

Then you are less likely to go back to the room and reopen the container for more. Even if you do, you burned extra calories and got extra steps by having to go back to the kitchen.

- *Add spice to your food.* Spices that help boost your metabolism and curb your hunger include cayenne pepper, black pepper, turmeric, cinnamon, and curry. Cayenne pepper, for instance, has been shown to help the body burn more fat when eaten with high-carb meals.

- *Consume more omega-3 fatty acids.* The hormone leptin, which causes a sensation of fullness after eating, is increased by the omega-3 fatty acids contained in fish, making them especially effective at lowering appetite.

- *Do not chew gum regularly or for extended periods of time.* The act of mastication (chewing) tells your body that food is on the way, so it speeds digestion up and makes you hungrier sooner than you otherwise may have been. For breath freshening, sip mint herbal teas or try the breath strips or sprays.

- *Pay attention to your urges for snacks.* If you ignore your hunger, it's possible that you'll overeat when it's time for a meal, which will make your hunger worse. Choose healthy options like hummus, carrot sticks, fruit, etc. whenever you feel like nibbling so you can help keep yourself full without consuming a lot of calories. If you are watching your macros, plan snacks that fit what you need for the day ahead of time. Then you can hit what your body needs, curb hunger before it hits, and not really have to give any time or thought to food on a daily basis- just once a week or so for planning time.

- *Sip on liquids to help you feel fuller longer.* Having a beverage with your meal may help you feel fuller with less food. Unfortunately, some individuals eat when they really need to drink water because they misinterpret their body's signals. That's less likely to occur if you drink plenty of water all throughout the day and with each meal.

- *Exercise is a great way to curb your appetite.* Exercise helps reduce your appetite by suppressing hunger hormones. Of course, you can't keep going if you don't give your body the nourishment it requires. A person's efforts to lose weight may backfire if they severely restrict their caloric intake and become too exhausted to keep up with their regular exercise routine. Therefore, the whole operation fails. Some of my patients have complained to me that physical activity just makes them hungrier and causes them to overeat. However, this is usually the result of inadequate pre- and post-workout nutrition.

- *Small, regular meals might help you control your hunger.* Eating modest, frequent meals throughout the day helps maintain more steady blood sugar levels. This is crucial since spikes in appetite can be brought on by drops in blood sugar. Even if you're worried that a smaller meal won't be enough to satisfy your hunger, knowing that you'll be able to refuel in a few hours could be extremely helpful. Others find that intermittent fasting is actually best for their body and hunger. Stay with me here, but for some not starting to eat for the day cause their appetite to not kick in yet. They report (and studies show) that intermittent fasting causes your body to burn your own fat stores when done properly. When you switch over to fat-burning mode, there is plenty of energy and no hunger. Some do intermittent as in 18 hours with no food, then 6 hours of eating or something equivalent. Others do 24 hr fasts weekly or bi-weekly.

- *Use dark chocolate to satisfy your sweet cravings.* Dark chocolate should be chosen over milk chocolate if you have a serious sweet tooth. When the cocoa content is 75% or 80% or above, there is less sugar and more room for moderation. Read research, talk with your doctor, and decide if "grazing" or intermittent fasting may be a better solution for your body and your lifestyle. Before you write them off, give them each a good try. You may be surprised at which one works best for your body. My favorite, as I mentioned earlier, is food cycling-a combination of the two. It seems to be a real plateau buster for most.

A Useful Method to Try

Okay, so let's say that you've followed every piece of advice I offered in this book, and now you have regular meals and maybe even scheduled snacks, or you are absolutely rocking intermittent fasting. During the first week of your new lifestyle, you may experience some mild symptoms, like hunger. Don't worry; this is typical. Because your body is still adapting to this new "normal," the first week or two of a new diet is usually the most difficult. Just remember to stick to your plan, and you won't just lose weight but also find that you're not as hungry as you were before after a few weeks. This is because you will be conditioning your body to anticipate meals only at certain times of day and in smaller amounts. However, the first two weeks may make or break a diet, so here's what I advise doing if those pesky hunger cues appear:

1. Drink

    Drinking 16 ounces of water (two cups) causes your stomach to expand, which signals your brain that you are no longer hungry. It's also ideal to consume these two cups at least 30 minutes before you plan to eat. This is because when you think about eating, your mouth starts to salivate and your stomach starts making digestive fluid to get ready for the meal. If you drink water just before eating in such a condition, your saliva and digestive secretions will dissolve. And since we already know that drinking water makes you feel full, you'll naturally consume fewer calories overall. You'll soon feel hungry again once the water has been absorbed, which might lead to overeating. Since most individuals mistake hunger for thirst, this approach is also helpful in determining whether you are indeed hungry. After drinking 16 ounces of water and waiting 15 minutes, you should find that your hunger pains have gone away. If they haven't, you're probably really hungry, in which case I recommend the next step.

2. Do Deep Breathing Exercises and Wait for 15 Minutes

To do breathing exercises, all you have to do is concentrate on your breathing while shutting off the world around you-easy, right? LOL. Deep breathing specifically is a kind of breathing exercise that entails taking a deep breath, holding it for a little while, and then slowly exhaling it. Every one of us has probably heard that regular breathing exercises help people relax, feel better, and concentrate more effectively. Because of this, it seems likely that doing breathing exercises regularly is good for mental health and, by extension, our quality of life. Fewer people, on the other hand, know how good it is for our physical health. When you train your breathing muscles on a daily basis, you not only improve your health but also reduce your appetite and increase your feelings of fullness. This helps you maintain a healthy weight by preventing you from eating too much. This impact of breathing exercises on appetite regulation was discovered in a study by (Voroshilov, 2017). The study specifically linked Qigong breathing exercises to improved appetite regulation. Qigong includes many ways to regulate appetite by bringing the body and mind into harmony. Standing is the best way to do the exercise, or modified standing with the body leaning forward and both upper limbs resting on a countertop. Ideally, standing upright with your feet shoulder-width apart and your hands either on your stomach or along the length of your body is the starting position. Draw your stomach in while taking a deep breath and straightening your shoulders. For three to four seconds, you should hold your breath while holding your stomach in and using your ab muscles to their fullest extent to retract your stomach muscles. As you exhale, your chest and abdominal muscles will relax, and your shoulders will return to their initial posture. At a minimum, you should do this exercise 10–15 times. If you are overweight and find it difficult to pull in your stomach while standing, you can perform this exercise while sitting and supporting yourself with both hands. While we're talking about the respiratory system, it's important to note that breathing with your diaphragm has been shown to speed up your metabolism. And because we all know that women in this stage of life have a slower metabolism, this may be the ideal solution for us gals over 40. This is brought on by the body's altered hormonal balance. That makes gaining weight much easier but losing weight much more difficult. This breathing method may help reduce stress eating, cortisol levels and aid in a quicker metabolism. Triple threat! In cases where the issue isn't how many calories you're consuming, calorie restriction won't always lead to weight reduction, but this breathing method may. This was demonstrated in a study by (Yong et al., 2018), in which half of the 38 participants engaged in diaphragmatic breathing. This is also called "belly breathing," and it means taking in enough air to stretch your diaphragm. The muscle that looks like a dome and is right above your stomach and below your lungs is called your diaphragm. The other half used feedback breathing devices to practice alternative breathing techniques. Researchers discovered a substantial difference in total oxygen intake and resting metabolic rate in the diaphragmatic breathing group. These benefits were not seen in the other group utilizing the breathing apparatus. The following is a guide for practicing diaphragmatic breathing:

- With your legs bent and a low pillow under your head, lie on your b- ' yoga mat or in bed. If m required, put a cushion beneath your knees.

- Put one hand slightly below your ribcage on your abdomen, and the other on your upper chest.

- Inhale deeply through your nose and feel the air settle into your torso and belly. At first, keep your hand motionless on your chest while raising your belly hand.

- As you gently exhale through pursed lips, tighten your abdominal muscles and allow them to go inward toward your spine. Return the hand to its previous position on your belly.

Spend at least 10 minutes a day using this breathing method to get more energy, a faster metabolism, lower blood pressure, and an easier time losing weight. Though it may take some extra work to get the hang of using your diaphragm properly at first, you'll quickly see the benefits of putting in the time and effort. Once you know how to do it, try it while sitting in a chair with your knees bent and your shoulders, head, and neck in a comfortable, neutral position, or you can just sit on your floor mat with your legs crossed as part of your yoga or other workout routines. Wait another 15 minutes after you've finished your breathing exercise before moving on to the next phase if hunger is still on your mind.

3. Eat a High Fiber Food

Pair a high-fiber food like celery with Pink Himalayan salt, or almond butter. Consume citrus fruits like oranges and grapefruits since they are high in soluble fiber and low in calories. These types of foods are fantastic for satiating appetites since they make us feel full more quickly and keep our blood sugar levels constant. I only propose oranges or grapefruit since they have the greatest fiber content among the top 20 fruits and vegetables, but it doesn't have to be those two. Oats, which are low in calories and have a lot of both soluble and insoluble fibers, are another good choice. The soluble fiber beta-glucan in oats keeps you feeling full for longer. This is one reason why oats are so popular as a breakfast food. A green salad would be a great choice as well since it's also very rich in fiber and you can top it with celery sticks. Celery sticks have a crunch that is comparable to that of chips or crackers, which makes them an excellent snack in general. Celery is also rich in water content, low in calories, and high in fiber. Now Include some Pink Himalayan salt for flavor and to increase its appetite-suppressing effects. Historically, Himalayan salt has been used in both Ayurvedic and TCM treatments. It has become popular in many health communities because of the health benefits it is said to have during intermittent fasting, such as more energy and a smoother digestive system. By increasing blood flow to your stomach, pink salt reduces hunger sensations by decreasing the amount of blood that travels there. Alternatively, if you don't want to eat more salt, I suggest adding a tiny bit of almond butter. Almond butter has a decent quantity of fiber and healthy fats, which may help you feel fuller for longer. You won't feel the need for a snack in between meals since it helps control your appetite. This is useful if you're trying to control or lose weight and are spacing out your meals and keeping an eye on your food consumption.

The Recap

Yay, you've made it to this part of the book! I am a gal who does not like to waste time-mine or anyone else's, so I wanted this book to have a quick reference section with just the bullet points of the important stuff. You've read the studies and digested the details (pun intended), now here is the "meat and potatoes" of how-to. Okay so first thing is water, the following should help:

Put Some Flavor in It

If you don't like the way water tastes or if you find drinking water dull, this is a fantastic alternative. Mix some fruit into your water. Citrus fruits like oranges, lemons, and limes have already been tried and tested-delish! Some more tasty alternatives are cucumbers, watermelons, berries, and mint. These can also make the drink pretty, and thus more fun to drink!

Eat It

Melons, cucumbers, lettuce, and celery are just a few examples of the many fruits and vegetables that are mostly composed of water, which makes it simpler to consume more water without realizing it. There are also a variety of soups, popsicles (though be careful with the sugar content), and smoothies to choose from (again watch the sugar here.)

Incorporate It Into Your Daily Schedule

Every time you clean your teeth, before you eat a meal, or before you enter the kitchen, drink a glass of water. One might find this approach to be very helpful. Because of this, I've been drinking a lot more water, and it has improved so much more than just my weight. I can't remember the last time my skin looked this glowy!

Follow It

The best way to keep track of your water intake is with a smart water bottle that syncs with your phone. Alternatively, you could use a calendar or alarm to keep tabs on your consumption.

Vary Your Beverage Choices

If you can't give up sugary drinks totally, try diluting them with water. When you've had enough water for the day, drink some soda or juice instead as a rare treat.

Grab It and Go

When you're always on the go, it might be hard to remember to take in enough fluids, therefore if you want to stay hydrated throughout the day, fill up a water bottle before you leave the house and carry it with you everywhere you go.

The Best Way to Kickstart Your Food Journaling Journey

Be gentle with yourself as you adapt, and try to be as consistent as you can. It's likely to be effective if it seems tough yet doable. Don't worry yourself sick if you miss a day here and there. Simply pick it back up right away. Just remember that this is a temporary state and it too shall pass. Keeping a food diary for a year or just today might teach you a lot about your eating habits. While the tried-and-true method of using a pen and piece of paper is still viable, it may not be for you. Take some images, use an app, or try writing something down on your phone to find the best option for you. That being said here are some tips I find useful for those new to journaling:

1. Don't Leave Anything Out of Your Record, Even if It's "Only a Taste."

    Even if you record every single meal and snack you have, your food diary won't be accurate if you don't also record the little, unnoticed bites of food and drink you have. Here are some examples, Say You're making dinner for the entire family, and you keep tasting it as you go to make sure it's not too salty or too sweet. Or, every time you pass by the office cafeteria, you swipe for a sweet dessert, or when you'd normally drink black coffee, but you choose to add creamer and sugar today. Note these events as they happen to ensure that your efforts are in line with your objectives, such as weight reduction or muscle building. Writing it down on the notes app on your phone and transferring it later to your diary is also an excellent strategy. These types of minor tastes are rather simple to quantify. If you decide to add half-and-half to your coffee, for instance, you may base your entry on the fact that one tablespoon of half-and-half has 20 calories. Write down your estimate of how much more you poured. In the grand scheme of things, the extra 20 calories from coffee cream won't matter, but if you're always nibbling and not recording, your diary will become inaccurate, and you'll be left wondering why you haven't accomplished your objectives.

2. Recognize Serving Sizes

For the first several weeks of keeping a food diary, you should measure meals exactly if you are unfamiliar with serving sizes. If you've never kept a food diary before, it's a good idea to get a food scale so you don't accidentally under-or overestimate your portions. All you need is an affordable food scale that you can get from the grocery store or a simple scale from Target. Eventually, you'll be able to forgo measuring cups and spoons in favor of winging it. Example: A deck of cards is roughly the same size as three ounces of protein. A ping pong ball is roughly the size of a two-tablespoon dollop of nut butter. The size of a teaspoon is comparable to a dice.

3. Give Detailed, Honest Information

Don't try to sugarcoat (I'm so punny) or otherwise alter what you ate in order to avoid feeling guilty; instead, record it precisely as it happened. For instance, don't be cheeky and simply type "potato" if you had fried chips. You'll go nowhere in the long term because this is too vague and lacks specificity. The terms "potato" and "fried chips" have quite distinct macronutrient profiles, so using them interchangeably won't help you monitor your nutrition.

4. Record the three Ws, including who, where, and when.

When did you eat, where did you eat, and who was there with you when you did? Our food consumption and dietary preferences are profoundly affected by all of these factors. Personally, I know that when I eat while watching TV, I consume much more calories than when I eat while seated at the table. It's possible that this is the case because I feel more at ease on the sofa since it's a less formal atmosphere and I can just chill. But I also know that I tend to overeat when I am in the company of others, most likely because I am too preoccupied with conversing and enjoying the company of others to notice that I am eating.

5. Snap Pictures

With our busy lives, the human memory isn't always as impressive as it could be. We are scattered and fragmented on a daily basis. You can easily fool yourself into believing a falsehood since our mental file cabinets are very prone to errors and forgetfulness. For this reason, it's recommended that, in addition to recording your meals in a diary, you also take photographs of them. Pictures tell a thousand words, plus it's always interesting to go back and examine how one's eating habits have changed over time.

Here Are Some Pointers for Maintaining a Regular Exercise Schedule

- **Aim for Something**

    Prioritize setting short-term objectives before moving on to longer-term ones. Ensure that your objectives are doable and realistic. If your objectives are too lofty, it'll be easy to lose motivation and give up. In the event that you haven't worked out in a while, a reasonable short-term objective may be to stroll for 10 minutes, five days a week. Of course, exercise, no matter how brief, has advantages. Aiming to get in 30 minutes of walking five days a week is a reasonable intermediate step. To walk five kilometers (~3 miles) would be a worthy long-term objective.

- **Make It Enjoyable**

    If you want to stay motivated, it's important to choose an activity or sport that you like doing and then mix it up. Exercise should be fun, so if you're not having fun, you should switch things up. Try out for a local softball or volleyball team. Learn some ballroom dance moves. Try visiting a nearby gym or dojo (or krav maga studio). You can find recordings of many other sorts of workout courses, including yoga, HIIT, and kickboxing, online if you want to work out in the comfort of your own home. Alternatively, you may go for a jog or a stroll at a nearby park. Learn about any latent sports hobbies or skills you may possess. Exercise need not be monotonous, and if you like it, you are more likely to persist with a fitness program.

- **Document It**

    Put your objectives on paper. If you can clearly see yourself reaping the benefits of regular exercise and write down your goals, you may find it easier to stay motivated. Keeping an exercise journal could just be what you were missing. Maintain a journal detailing your workouts, how long they lasted, and how you felt afterward. Keeping a log of your efforts and accomplishments might encourage you to keep pushing forward toward your objectives.

- **Include Exercise in Your Everyday Regimen**

    Finding time to exercise might be challenging, but that's no reason to put it off. To be effective, physical exercise must be planned ahead of time, just like any other mandatory task. Regular exercise can be integrated into your day in little increments. For example, Rather than using the elevator, make it a thing to start using the steps instead. Or as you watch the children play sports, stroll up and down the sidelines. Get some fresh air and exercise during your company's break time by going for a stroll, etc. It's especially important for those who work from home to take frequent breaks to get up and move about. Alternatively, you can perform sit-ups, lunges, and squats. Go for a walk with your dog if you have one.

Spend your lunch break or evenings in front of the TV doing some strength training routines, such as pedaling a stationary bike or walking/jogging on a treadmill. While doing the necessary amount of exercise each week is important for good health, studies show that sitting for lengthy periods of time might have a detrimental impact on health. If your profession requires you to sit for long periods of time, try to include short periods of movement throughout your day. This might be as simple as getting up to grab a sip of water or as involved as standing up during phone calls or online conferences.

- **Treat Yourself**

Make sure you allow yourself some time after each workout to bask in the glow of satisfaction. Motivating yourself in this way might help you maintain your fitness routine over time. Other incentives may also be good. Reward yourself with a new pair of walking shoes or some new music to listen to as you walk after you meet a long-term fitness goal.

- **Be Adaptable**

  If you're sick, overworked, or just plain tired, you're allowed to skip a day or two from your usual regimen. Relax your standards if you feel like you need a break without criticizing yourself too harshly. The most crucial thing anyway is to quickly resume your original course of action as soon as you can. Get going after your energy has returned! Set your own objectives, have fun with it, and sometimes give yourself a pat on the back. Never underestimate the value of exercise. If you find your drive waning again, revisit these suggestions.

How to Get Motivated to Start Working When You're Having Mental Issues

For good reason, the adage "getting started is the hardest part" is often used. The motivation needed to start any endeavor might be far higher than the motivation needed to complete it after you've gained momentum and concentration, whether it's exercising, regularly writing, attempting to control your emotional eating, etc. Even the most basic actions, like remembering to drink water or maintaining your resolve and resisting the urge to go for that muffin, may seem plain hard if you are also feeling anxious or cognitively challenged that day. Fortunately, the advice I provided you in the chapters above on how to deal with stress or emotional upheaval should be able to help you out sufficiently. However, I just wanted to give a brief refresher and a few more tips on how to make your first week a little bit easier. So, If you're having difficulties getting things done, whether it's your to-do list or your day-to-day obligations, try one of these methods to rekindle your drive.

Make A Plan. Work The Plan

Having a pile of unorganized tasks to complete staring you in the face is a certain way to put you in a funk and make whatever issue you're already facing much more difficult to handle. In such a scenario, time management is crucial. You should sit down for a period of time each day, and document/organize before starting the everyday activities. (Or do this once per week for the whole week). Exercise in the morning, complete important tasks in the first three hours so that you can rest after your workday is through, take a stroll around your building at lunch to get some fresh air, and so on are some examples. Whatever way you choose to organize it, be sure to reserve certain times of the day for certain duties. Making a schedule for your day helps you feel a lot more in control of your responsibilities. You may use your phone's calendar with notifications to remind you when to switch tasks, or a specific app.

Take Everything Step-By-Step

To avoid feeling overwhelmed, break down each item on your list into smaller, ostensibly more manageable chores. You'll get a dopamine rush as you check each item off the list. I promise you'll feel great about yourself for getting things done like when you do all the exercises you set out to do in a single session or refrain from overeating. By breaking up longer tasks into shorter bursts, you can get a lot done. Although it won't last long, this impact will provide you with just enough motivation to get you through those times when you're not feeling driven. No matter how much you may believe you are capable of, it is easier to motivate yourself when you have little, short tasks to do.

Compile an Inspiring Playlist

Lots of individuals, including myself, have a go-to playlist for when we need to buckle down and get through a tough endeavor. Certain types of music have the ability to truly motivate you to take action. It might be easier to be in the correct frame of mind and even feel more at ease when you're feeling off, uninspired, or just plain worried if your work area has a regular background. If you have a favorite playlist, whether it's one you made yourself or one you found on Spotify or YouTube, it's best to stick to it. Put in some fresh tunes every so often to keep things interesting.

Don an Attractive Outfit

This may sound strange, vain, or superficial, but there is truth to it. Clothing and accessories may help you feel more confident and put together when you're feeling overwhelmed by life's stresses. Putting on an item of clothing that makes you feel really good about yourself may be a great confidence booster. Even if you don't feel like working out today, putting on some nice exercise attire will help spark some enthusiasm. Wake up, get up, dress up, show up.

Conclusion

So, to recap and leave you with knowledge, empowerment, and encouragement: As we get older, it gets harder to keep weight off for a variety of reasons, such as stress, hormones, a slower metabolism, and so on. Even so, that doesn't mean that nothing can be done about it. The goal of this book was to show you how to lose weight after age 40 in a healthy way. I intended to demonstrate weight loss and weight maintenance FACTS, which is why the chapters were labeled as they were. I wanted the book to leave you with a sense of optimism and hope, not simply instructions for doing the thing. Instead of becoming disheartened, I want you to rise to the challenge by using the simple strategies offered in this book. I want you to accept that this is NOT your new normal and do something about it. You may have thought that there's no hope for regaining the weight-loss success you had at age 25, but if you're willing to put in the effort and follow a good strategy, you won't have to worry about your weight again. Whether your goal is to increase your water intake, raise your level of self-awareness, increase your daily step count, or increase your vegetable consumption, the key is to simply get started and keep going. Humans are hardwired to respond more strongly to negative feelings like self-doubt and self-pity, but I can promise you that these are merely your cavewoman brain's attempt to keep you feeling "secure" and comfortable. When you hear it, tell it to get lost and remind yourself, "I can do anything I put my mind to!" because, well, you are amazing! Now that you're equipped with this knowledge and revved up, there's no better time to start.

Share Your Experience!

I hope you're finding the strategies and insights in this book both practical and inspiring as you work towards your weight loss goals. Your journey is incredibly important, and I'm honored to be a part of it.

At this point in the book, you've likely had the opportunity to explore several tips and techniques that could make a real difference in your life. If you've found this book helpful, I'd love to hear from you!

Why Reviews Matter:

Your feedback is invaluable. By sharing your thoughts on Amazon, you help others who are seeking guidance on their own weight loss journeys. Your review can offer a glimpse into how this book has impacted you, and it can inspire others to take their first steps toward a healthier lifestyle.

How to Leave a Review:

1. **Visit the Book's Amazon Page**:
   https://www.amazon.com/review/review-

your-purchases/?asin=B0D3ZK83X4

2. **Share Your Thoughts**: Whether it's a brief note about what you've found most useful or an overview of your experience, your insights will be greatly appreciated.
3. **Rate the Book**: If you've found the content beneficial, a five-star rating helps others find this resource more easily.

Your honest feedback not only helps me improve but also supports the wider community of readers looking for effective weight loss solutions.

Thank you so much for your time and support. I'm thrilled to be part of your journey and excited to hear about your experiences!

Love,

Dr. Amanda Borre, D.C.

References

Berg, J. (2021, August 31). Tamra Judge Is Done with the Keto Diet: *"I gained weight."* Bravo TV Official Site; Bravo. https://www.bravotv.com/the-real-housewives-of-orange-county/style-living/tamra-judge-stops-keto-diet-after-weight-gain

Boschmann, M., Steiniger, J., Hille, U., Tank, J., Adams, F., Sharma, A. M., Klaus, S., Luft, F. C., & Jordan, J. (2003, December 1). *Water-induced Thermogenesis*. The Journal of Clinical Endocrinology & Metabolism, 88(12), 6015–6019. https://doi.org/10.1210/jc.2003-030780

Brown, C. M., Dulloo, A. G., & Montani, J.-P. (2006, September 1). Water-Induced Thermogenesis Reconsidered: *The effects of Osmolality and water temperature on energy expenditure after drinking*. The Journal of Clinical Endocrinology & Metabolism, 91(9), 3598–3602. https://doi.org/10.1210/jc.2006-0407

Castro-Sepulveda, M., Ramirez-Campillo, R., Abad-Colil, F., Monje, C., Peñailillo, L., Cancino, J., & Zbinden-Foncea, H. (2018, September 26). *Basal mild dehydration increase salivary cortisol after a friendly match in young elite soccer players*. Frontiers in

Physiology, 9. https://doi.org/10.3389/fphys.2018.01347

Corney, R. A., Sunderland, C., & James, L. J. (2015, April 18). *Immediate pre-meal water ingestion decreases voluntary food intake in lean young males*. European Journal of Nutrition, 55(2), 815–819. https://doi.org/10.1007/s00394-015-0903-4

Davy, B. M., Dennis, E. A., Dengo, A. L., Wilson, K. L., & Davy, K. P. (2008, July). *Water Consumption Reduces Energy Intake at a Breakfast Meal in Obese Older Adults*. Journal of the American Dietetic Association, 108(7), 1236–1239. https://doi.org/10.1016/j.jada.2008.04.013

Dehghan, M., Mente, A., Zhang, X., Swaminathan, S., Li, W., Mohan, V., Iqbal, R., Kumar, R., Wentzel-Viljoen, E., Rosengren, A., Amma, L. I., Avezum, A., Chifamba, J., Diaz, R., Khatib, R., Lear, S., Lopez-Jaramillo, P., Liu, X., Gupta, R., & Mohammadifard, N. (2017, November 04). Associations of fats and carbohydrate intake with cardiovascular disease and mortality in 18 countries from five continents (PURE): *a prospective cohort study*. The Lancet, 390(10107), 2050–2062. https://doi.org/10.1016/s0140-6736(17)32252-3

Donnelly, J. E., Honas, J. J., Smith, B. K., Mayo, M. S., Gibson, C. A., Sullivan, D. K., Lee, J., Herrmann, S. D., Lambourne, K., & Washburn, R. A. (2013, March 21). Aerobic exercise alone results in clinically significant weight loss for men and women: *Midwest exercise trial 2*. Obesity, 21(3),

E219–E228. https://doi.org/10.1002/oby.20145

Garcia-Navarro, L. (2018, April 29). "Tully Gets It": *Charlize Theron Wants An Honest Conversation About Motherhood.* NPR.org. https://www.npr.org/2018/04/29/606062105/tully-gets-it-charlize-theron-wants-an-honest-conversation-about-motherhood

Harland, J. I., & Garton, L. E. (2008a, June 11). *Whole-grain intake as a marker of healthy body weight and adiposity.* Public Health Nutrition, 11(6), 554–563. https://doi.org/10.1017/s1368980007001279

Harland, J. I., & Garton, L. E. (2008b, June 11). *Whole-grain intake as a marker of healthy body weight and adiposity.* Public Health Nutrition, 11(6), 554–563. https://doi.org/10.1017/s1368980007001279

Hollis, J. F., Gullion, C. M., Stevens, V. J., Brantley, P. J., Appel, L. J., Ard, J. D., Champagne, C. M., Dalcin, A., Erlinger, T. P., Funk, K., Laferriere, D., Lin, P.-H., Loria, C. M., Samuel-Hodge, C., Vollmer, W. M., & Svetkey, L. P. (2008a, August). *Weight Loss During the Intensive Intervention Phase of the Weight-Loss Maintenance Trial.* American Journal of Preventive Medicine, 35(2), 118–126. https://doi.org/10.1016/j.amepre.2008.04.013

Hollis, J. F., Gullion, C. M., Stevens, V. J., Brantley, P. J., Appel, L. J., Ard, J. D., Champagne, C. M.,

Dalcin, A., Erlinger, T. P., Funk, K., Laferriere, D., Lin, P.-H., Loria, C. M., Samuel-Hodge, C., Vollmer, W. M., & Svetkey, L. P. (2008b, August). *Weight Loss During the Intensive Intervention Phase of the Weight-Loss Maintenance Trial.* American Journal of Preventive Medicine, 35(2), 118–126.
https://doi.org/10.1016/j.amepre.2008.04.013

Hollis, J. F., Gullion, C. M., Stevens, V. J., Brantley, P. J., Appel, L. J., Ard, J. D., Champagne, C. M., Dalcin, A., Erlinger, T. P., Funk, K., Laferriere, D., Lin, P.-H., Loria, C. M., Samuel-Hodge, C., Vollmer, W. M., & Svetkey, L. P. (2008c, August). *Weight Loss During the Intensive Intervention Phase of the Weight-Loss Maintenance Trial.* American Journal of Preventive Medicine, 35(2), 118–126.
https://doi.org/10.1016/j.amepre.2008.04.013

How Habits Work - Charles Duhigg. (2017, November 20). Charles Duhigg.
https://charlesduhigg.com/how-habits-work/

Longland, T. M., Oikawa, S. Y., Mitchell, C. J., Devries, M. C., & Phillips, S. M. (2016, January 27). *Higher compared with lower dietary protein during an energy deficit combined with intense exercise promotes greater lean mass gain and fat mass loss: a randomized trial.* The American Journal of Clinical Nutrition, 103(3), 738–746.
https://doi.org/10.3945/ajcn.115.119339

Madjd, A., Taylor, M. A., Delavari, A., Malekzadeh, R., Macdonald, I. A., & Farshchi, H. R. (2015,

November 4). Effects on weight loss in adults of replacing diet beverages with water during a hypoenergetic diet: *a randomized, 24-wk clinical trial.* The American Journal of Clinical Nutrition, 102(6), 1305–1312. https://doi.org/10.3945/ajcn.115.109397

Morita, Yokoyama, Imai, Takeda, Ota, Kawai, Hisada, Emoto, Suzuki, & Okazaki. (2019a, April 17). *Aerobic Exercise Training with Brisk Walking Increases Intestinal Bacteroides in Healthy Elderly Women.* Nutrients, 11(4), 868. https://doi.org/10.3390/nu11040868

Morita, Yokoyama, Imai, Takeda, Ota, Kawai, Hisada, Emoto, Suzuki, & Okazaki. (2019b, April 17). *Aerobic Exercise Training with Brisk Walking Increases Intestinal Bacteroides in Healthy Elderly Women.* Nutrients, 11(4), 868. https://doi.org/10.3390/nu11040868

News-Medical. (2019, September 25). *Americans still eat too many low-quality carbs and saturated fats, say experts.* News-Medical.net. https://www.news-medical.net/news/20190925/Americans-still-eat-too-many-low-quality-carbs-and-saturated-fats-say-experts.aspx

Paddock, C. (2015, July 13). *Americans "not eating enough fruits and vegetables."* Medicalnewstoday.com; Medical News Today.

https://www.medicalnewstoday.com/articles/296677

Quinn, C. (2016, August 12). *A Simple Strategy That'll Make You Drink More Water Every Day*. Thrillist; Thrillist. https://www.thrillist.com/health/nation/hydration-tips-to-drink-more-water-every-day

Shan, Z., Rehm, C. D., Rogers, G., Ruan, M., Wang, D. D., Hu, F. B., Mozaffarian, D., Zhang, F. F., & Bhupathiraju, S. N. (2019, September 24). *Trends in Dietary Carbohydrate, Protein, and Fat Intake and Diet Quality Among US Adults, 1999-2016*. JAMA, 322(12), 1178. https://doi.org/10.1001/jama.2019.13771

Sondike, S. B., Copperman, N., & Jacobson, M. S. (2003, March). *Effects of a low-carbohydrate diet on weight loss and cardiovascular risk factor in overweight adolescents*. The Journal of Pediatrics, 142(3), 253–258. https://doi.org/10.1067/mpd.2003.4

Stookey, J. D., Constant, F., Popkin, B. M., & Gardner, C. D. (2008, November 16). *Drinking Water Is Associated With Weight Loss in Overweight Dieting Women Independent of Diet and Activity*. Obesity, 16(11), 2481–2488. https://doi.org/10.1038/oby.2008.409

Tantawy, S., Kamel, D., Abdel-Basset, W., & Elgohary, H. (2017a, December 14). *Effects of a proposed physical activity and diet control to manage constipation in middle-aged obese women*. Diabetes, Metabolic Syndrome and Obesity: Targets and Therapy,

Volume 10, 513–519. https://doi.org/10.2147/dmso.s140250

Tantawy, S., Kamel, D., Abdel-Basset, W., & Elgohary, H. (2017b, December 14). *Effects of a proposed physical activity and diet control to manage constipation in middle-aged obese women.* Diabetes, Metabolic Syndrome and Obesity: Targets and Therapy, Volume 10, 513–519. https://doi.org/10.2147/dmso.s140250

The technique that will allow us to change the habits we do not like (Charles Duhigg) | Part B' (2022, January 21). Lectures Bureau. https://www.lecturesbureau.gr/1/the-technique-that-will-allow-us-to-change-the-habits-we-do-not-like-part-b-2818b/?lang=en

Thornton, S. N. (2016, June 10). *Increased Hydration Can Be Associated with Weight Loss.* Frontiers in Nutrition, 3. https://doi.org/10.3389/fnut.2016.00018

Vij, V. A. (2013, September 7). *Effect of "Water Induced Thermogenesis" on Body Weight, Body Mass Index and Body Composition of Overweight Subjects.* Journal of Clinical and Diagnostic Research. https://doi.org/10.7860/jcdr/2013/5862.3344

Voroshilov, A. P. (2017, May 12). *Modified Qigong breathing exercise for reducing the sense of hunger on an empty stomach* - Alexander P. Voroshilov, Alex A. Volinsky, Zhixin Wang, Elena V. Marchenko, 2017. Journal of Evidence-Based Complementary & Alternative Medicine.

https://journals.sagepub.com/doi/10.1177/2156587217707143#:~:text=The%20Modified%20Qigong%20Breathing%20Exercise&text=Hold%20your%20breath%20for%203,Repeat%20this%20exercise%2010%20times.

Weigle. (2005, July). *A high-protein diet induces sustained reductions in appetite, ad libitum caloric intake, and body weight despite compensatory changes in diurnal plasma leptin and ghrelin concentrations.* The American Journal of Clinical Nutrition, 82(1). https://doi.org/10.1093/ajcn.82.1.41

Wempen, K. (2022, April 29). *Are you getting too much protein?* Mayo Clinic Health System; Mayo Clinic Health System. https://www.mayoclinichealthsystem.org/hometown-health/speaking-of-health/are-you-getting-too-much-protein

Yong, M.-S., Lee, Y.-S., & Lee, H.-Y. (2018a, September 30). *Effects of breathing exercises on resting metabolic rate and maximal oxygen uptake.* Journal of Physical Therapy Science, 30(9), 1173–1175. https://doi.org/10.1589/jpts.30.1173

Yong, M.-S., Lee, Y.-S., & Lee, H.-Y. (2018b, September 30). Effects of breathing exercises on resting metabolic rate and maximal oxygen uptake. Journal of Physical Therapy Science, 30(9), 1173–1175. https://doi.org/10.1589/jpts.30.1173

Section 2:
5 Fast Flat Belly Facts

Introduction

A flat tummy: The secret weapon to a healthy life.
—Best Slogans, n.d.

Ever since I came across this phrase, I have not been able to stop thinking about how powerful it is! Time and again, we have been told how our body weight affects our overall health. An excessive increase or decrease in weight is typically an alarming indication of various underlying health conditions. Yet, throughout the decades, society's conception of aesthetics has depended a lot on a person's weight and size. From beauty pageants to the movies, slim people are portrayed as appealing and beautiful. The good news is that many of these superficial beauty standards all across the globe are shifting, and I'm delighted to live in an era where individuals have started focusing on their uniqueness, self-love, and self-expression. This is a source of hope for me and undoubtedly for many others like me.

However, from a medical point of view, we cannot deny that gaining too much weight can lead to a myriad of health issues. Obesity and the accumulation of visceral fat—or belly fat—are some of the leading causes of serious health conditions, such as cardiovascular diseases, high blood pressure, certain cancers, stroke, gallstones, diabetes, and many more. So, while being overweight or having excessive fat density is not necessarily an aesthetic concern, it should not be neglected because it adds to the risk factors for your health. Maintaining a healthy weight is vital to preventing and controlling several conditions and diseases.

You've probably heard that as you get older, you are more likely to gain weight or add inches around your belly and other portions of your body. Your metabolism—which is mostly in charge of managing your body's weight—functions significantly differently or, rather, a bit slower as you get older. And while this is true, you shouldn't use it as an excuse to give up on your efforts to get healthy. Get after it! You *can* make a change!

Given our hectic lifestyles, the hustle and bustle of daily life, and the jobs and commitments that hang over us all, it makes sense that you might feel like you don't have enough time to pause and evaluate your overall well-being. However, these conditions are an inevitable aspect of life, and we can't downplay the significance of maintaining good health and fitness in the light of advancing years and stressful situations. Your health should always be a priority—no matter what.

According to research, "Most of the world's population live in countries where overweight and obesity kill more people than underweight" (World Health Organization, 2021). Obesity and being overweight are conditions where there is an overabundance of fat in the body, which can cause severe health damage. So, your waistline has a lot to do with your overall health, and a lot of us are in trouble. I say we turn these statistics around.

Doctors emphasize the fact that the fat around the belly is the most dangerous of all types of fat. This is because the accumulation of such fat starts in the abdominal region and gradually spreads into other organs (Lemos, 2020).

Fat content is always present in the human body. However, the problem arises when there is an imbalance in the amount and type of fat deposit. For instance, the fat that lies immediately under your skin is called subcutaneous fat. You can feel this type of fat by pinching your skin. Visceral fat, on the other hand, is found in your intestines and stomach areas. Visceral fat is mostly responsible for the formation of various ailments in your body.

Research also shows that larger waist size can be a huge concern—for women, more than 35 inches, and for men, more than 40 inches (Wade, 2015). This is a prime reason why it's necessary to shed extra fat around the belly to stay fit in the long run.

Abdominal obesity is strongly linked to various health conditions. So, losing or, rather, reaching a healthy weight and size can have tremendous advantages to your holistic health. Here are some of the most important reasons why having a healthy body and a flat tummy is so crucial for everyone, regardless of age or gender:

- A healthy BMI and a flatter tummy can help prevent many diseases. Abdominal obesity is associated with a high risk of cardiovascular diseases, hypertension, type 2 diabetes, asthma, sleep apnea, Alzheimer's disease, and insulin resistance. Also, with an increase in the waist and hip ratio, there is a greater chance of developing conditions such as blood lipid disorders, metabolic syndrome, and various other physical ailments (Westphal, 2008).

- The size of your waist can also be related to knee osteoarthritis. Obese people are more likely to experience aches, which can have a severe impact on their flexibility and mobility. A flatter tummy can make you feel healthier and also help you stay active and swift for a longer time. Visceral fat plays a strong role in affecting your body's functioning, and by reducing it, you can stay fit and healthy. Simply put, visceral fat helps produce cytokines, an inflammatory chemical, which can cause inflammation and lead to autoimmune and neurodegenerative diseases (Wade, 2015).

- Health is not only about your physical condition; it is also about your mental state. Research shows that excessive fat in the abdomen can adversely affect cognitive functions (Dolan, 2023). By keeping a check on the growing fat around your midsection and your overall weight, you can help prevent many diseases caused by lifestyle issues. Obesity can also play a major role in how you operate in your day-to-day life. From self-esteem issues and difficulty conducting regular activities to developing life-threatening diseases, your growing weight and size can cause serious disruptions to your normal routine. Your physical *and* mental health can benefit from working toward a more fit and healthy life.

I think you'll agree with me when I say that weight gain is tricky to understand. For example, you might be eating healthy and working out daily, but you simply cannot lose any weight. Contrary to popular belief, consuming more food is not the only thing that results in weight gain. In fact, weight gain can result from a variety of factors. Hormonal imbalance, sugar and sodium consumption, medications, certain health conditions, and not having a well-rounded diet can lead to a higher accumulation of fat and an increase in your overall weight.

Let me share an interesting thing I recently came across while scrolling through a social media page. Edna, a middle-aged, plus-sized woman, lost 20 pounds in only a couple of weeks. When I came across this video, I started watching, feeling curious, interested, and quite inspired until toward the end, she pulled out a package of some "magic" tea bags and showed it to the viewers. As a wellness and health fanatic, I was taken aback when I heard her say she lost a considerable amount of body fat and dramatically reduced her weight by simply sipping the "tea" for a month and doing nothing more! By the time I could fully understand that this was a commercial that only looked like a person genuinely telling her story, I had already started to feel uneasy about how the weight-loss industry has taken the world by storm—in quite an adverse way!

I find it unfortunate that we live in an age when there is nearly unlimited access to information, but it is a challenge to figure out what is genuine and what is not. These days, the market is mostly digitized and relies on marketing techniques that only look real to customers. In the case of Edna, I was hooked on the video and was interested right until the end, when I figured out what she "did" to make her weight vanish in only a few days. And while the medical professional in me found it appalling and unrealistic, I cannot deny that I was watching the video very attentively. This type of marketing is part of the real problem and can be very dangerous in the long term. I realized that there must be millions like me watching the video, and many of them were probably buying what she was selling!

That's how business works, right? But, seriously, I am not up for it! It was then that I decided to make a real effort to bring the truth to people trying to lose weight. I became determined to help them achieve their goals by guiding them in the most practical and healthiest way possible. From a health and medical point of view, I fully understand the disadvantages of gaining weight (and more so, visceral fat). Your health is important, so what you use on and in your body has to be "marked safe" before using it—because even a small glitch can make you suffer.

Just like a parent strives to give the best possible advice and the finest quality food to their children, please realize that you have to be equally wary about your own health and fitness. If weight loss and shedding a few inches from your belly is your goal, then your priority should also be turning to the most authentic ways to get there. Don't depend on fad diets and tricks that seldom work and also have probable side effects. Join me on this journey where we dig into the treasure trove of knowledge that will help you gain an understanding of how your body operates.

We all have ideas about how we can lose weight, but there are specific aspects we need to look into further. First, it is essential to comprehend the root causes of weight gain. Yes, every time you look in the mirror and see a slight double chin peeking out or pull on a pair of jeans that suddenly seem a little too tight, such can be your body's way of telling you that you are weighing in a bit more than usual. And while the physical aspects of weight issues are visible, we also need to address the unseen psychological aspects.

Unfortunately, societal pressures and stereotypical judgments based on a person's weight often outweigh (pun intended) many other beautiful features they possess. Many people today—maybe even you!—still measure their worth through the weight on a scale. Let me set this straight: Your weight does not define you! My whole point is to make you understand that losing weight should never be about how others perceive you or how much you want them to approve of you. It has to be with only one perspective—and that is to improve your health and lead a long, vital life.

If you think about it, when you were younger, you could run up the stairs and not pant. With age or with a few extra pounds, it could get difficult to even take the stairs up to the second floor, let alone run! This is what fitness is about; the stubborn weight or a growing belly can make you feel exhausted and unwell and even dwindle your self-esteem at times. While some people recognize these problems and work on them right away, others might feel like they can't do anything due to a lack of time, focus, or even a sense of guilt about taking care of themselves. Taking a few minutes each day to work on yourself is not much to ask for; but I also understand that for many, it can be a huge challenge.

One solution to such situations is to understand your health inside and out and how it relates to your holistic well-being. You do not have to have a fancy gym membership or buy products that promise to trim your waist. All you have to do is stay with me until the end of this book, understand how our body works, and learn how you can use it to your benefit. We will talk about the top five ways to keep your weight, body fat, and, most importantly, your general well-being in the best shape possible. Through years of meticulous study and research, I have come up with interesting ways to understand why having a flat tummy is important and how you can achieve it by simply following a few methods.

You chose this book because something inside makes you think you need motivation and—most importantly—some guidance to achieve a certain fitness level demonstrated by a flatter stomach. Bravo for the decision you made to take a step forward and learn ways to feel and look better. You are already taking action by seeking help and reading to learn more. Here are a few areas you will have a better understanding of by the time you finish reading this book:

- **Your health matters.** This book is carefully crafted to help you understand how important your health is and how everything else revolves around it. It will boost your confidence as you read about every little detail of how your body works, inside and out. The more you get into the intricacies of your physical and mental health, you will be able to incorporate that knowledge into your weight loss and waist-reduction process.

- **Your food matters.** Most of the time, we think that losing weight and staying fit is about not eating as much, but with the help of the various topics covered in this book, you will get a clear picture of how food can affect your overall health. I'll cover the foods that can be helpful and the foods that can put you in danger to help you make smart and careful choices.

At the end of the day, this is how you can rediscover happiness with yourself. By revitalizing your inner strength and working things through intelligently, you'll be able to enjoy a fresh outlook and a newfound zeal.

The adage "Prevention is better than cure" sums up how taking care of your health at the right time can help you stay in good spirits and health for the rest of your life, and starting your fitness journey is not limited to a certain age, gender, or body type. Whatever stage of life you are in, taking steps to get healthy again is important. It doesn't matter if you are a student who feels overweight and uneasy, you are one of the busiest people around, you have recently recovered from a medical condition, or you are retired. All it takes to significantly enhance your quality of life is the will to work on yourself and the effort to make a few slight modifications to the way you live. In no time, you will feel the difference and come to meet the healthier version of yourself. There is no time like the present—so let's get started!

Chapter 1:

Sodium Sensitivity

On certain days, when you wake up in the morning, you may notice that your face feels puffier than usual. Well, in some cases, you can blame the delicious food you consumed the previous day. In a situation like this, you will notice that no amount of lymphatic drainage massages or gua sha can come to the rescue. Food with a high sodium content can be one of the biggest causes of water retention in your body, especially in your stomach.

As a teenager, I remember my brother and I poured salt into my mom's water glass on a vacation to the rodeo. She was so swollen, she couldn't get her boots off! We thought we were *hilarious*. Her? Not so much. Sodium sensitivity is real and can adversely affect your health in many ways.

Every time sodium is mentioned, most people tend to think about salt. Though not wrong, there is a slight difference in salt and sodium, which is quite interesting to understand. Sodium is a dietary mineral that is required for muscle and nerve functions and to balance the body's fluids and minerals. Salt, on the other hand, contains 40% sodium and 60% chloride (Harvard School of Public Health, 2019). Salt is also known as sodium chloride for this reason. We season our meals with table salt, which is mostly composed of sodium chloride. Simply put, sodium is present in salt.

In numerous cases, sodium sensitivity is referred to as salt sensitivity, which is a change in health condition mainly caused by an increase or decrease in sodium intake. Blood pressure is one of the major areas that is highly affected by sodium sensitivity issues. This can further lead to many medical complications and conditions, like hypertension, cardiovascular diseases, and even stroke. Understanding the role of sodium in your health and everything related to it can be one of the best ways to keep track of your nutrition and health conditions, as well as keep your waist trim.

Understanding Sodium Intake

The U.S. Food and Drug Administration (FDA) has made huge efforts to curb the excessive sodium contained in mostly packaged and processed foods. We consume about 70% of the sodium in our diets through packaged food. This is one of the reasons why keeping track of what you eat and the nutritional content of packaged food is very important (FDA, 2020). And while imagining a saltless diet can seem pretty boring, it is also true that the excessive sodium present in salt can be harmful. So, understanding sodium intake is very important for your health.

Recommended Daily Allowance

The average American consumes about 3,400 milligrams (mg) of sodium per day, which is more than double the federal recommendation (CDC, 2019). The American Heart Association recommends around 1,500 mg of sodium daily. However, a more practical goal is to not consume more than 2,300 mg of sodium each day (Creekside Family Practice, n.d.).

Sources of Hidden Sodium

Many times, people begin a low-sodium diet for medical and weight-loss reasons. They avoid known sodium, but despite their best efforts, they continue to experience concerns with bloating, water retention, and high blood pressure. Unknown sources of salt in your diet may also be a major contributing factor.

If you have experienced this, you might want to food journal to pinpoint potential causes. For instance, countless food items have sodium, which may not be easy to track unless you are journaling to look back at symptoms versus food intake. Here are a few food items that are some of the sneakiest places where sodium hides:

- sauces, like soy, oyster, Worcestershire, pasta, etc.

- canned foods, like soups, stews, and other food items

- seasoning, condiments, bouillon, ready-made pastes, meat tenderizers, and dressings for food and salads

- frozen meals with sauces and gravy

- processed and packaged food, like salted chips, popcorn, pretzels, crackers, pork rinds, biscuits, noodles, pasta, vegetables, sausages, nuggets, cereals, etc.

- cured, canned, and smoked meat and fish

- different types of cheese and deli meats

- ready-made mixes like pudding, cakes, etc.

- egg whites and cottage cheese (These are the two that surprised me most!)

Apart from these sneaky sodium items, you can even find sodium in small traces in several medicines. Consulting your medical practitioner regarding any of your medical conditions and medications can be a good way to understand what you are consuming.

Reading the back of nutrition labels is a great habit to get into for many reasons. Many times, items that are termed "low-calorie" or "low-sodium" may trick you into believing that there is very little to no sodium at all. However, it is always a good idea to be aware of what you are consuming by checking the details and labels of food products carefully.

Effects of Excessive Sodium

Have you recently experienced feeling excessively thirsty and bloated? This could be one or more of the symptoms of consuming excessive sodium! As we've already seen, there are countless types of food sources that might contain sodium, so keeping a check on the total amount in all the foods you are consuming regularly can be difficult.

If sodium is not taken in moderation or smaller amounts, this might result in a number of health issues as well. Here are some of the ways excessive sodium can affect you if you don't take control:

Water Retention and Bloating

Too much sodium can cause swelling in various parts of the body, mostly in the ankles, feet, legs, face, hands, and stomach. This condition is also known as edema, and it can also be influenced by many underlying health conditions that cause the tissues to accumulate more fluid than needed.

Studies have shown how an increase in sodium intake can cause bloating. According to the National Library of Medical Science, reducing sodium is a crucial dietary intervention that can help reduce bloating and other related symptoms (Peng et al., 2019).

There are days when you feel heavier than usual and particularly not at your best. The chances are you are facing some water retention issues in your system. Here are some signs and symptoms that could hint at this condition:

- swollen parts of the body, like a puffy face and feet
- bloating in the stomach and abdomen
- fluctuation in weight, like sudden weight gain in only a few days
- reduced flexibility and stiff feeling in the joints
- visible indent forming when pressing on the swollen areas of the body
- body aches

Aside from sodium, there are many reasons why you might retain water, including long periods of traveling on flights, prolonged sitting or standing, health conditions, medications, pregnancy, menstruation, hormonal fluctuations, liver and kidney issues, etc.

Fluid retention can be classified into two categories: generalized edema and localized edema. In the first case, the entire body gets swollen, and in the second case, only specific body parts get swollen. As already mentioned, there could be many reasons for this, but a very common cause of mild water retention is excessive consumption of sodium or salt (Better Health Channel, 2012).

Regardless of what type of water retention you may be facing, it is very important to understand the real diagnosis or cause of the condition. Proper consultation with a doctor, physical tests, and investigating medical history are crucial to help prevent or cure any medical condition in the long run.

Here are a few strategies to help you significantly reduce water retention:

- **Swap out high-sodium foods:** Replace sodium-laden food sources with low-sodium foods or alternatives. Table salt is a source of sodium, but the hidden sodium content in many foods can be problematic. Almost 75% of the sodium consumed by most people comes not from cooking salt but from other unnoticed sources of food. Checking the quality and content of all food items before consumption is the best way to control sodium intake (Smith, 2023).

- **Drink more water:** Dehydration can cause the body to retain more fluid in the system, causing water retention issues. Drinking enough water is the best way to prevent this condition. It can also help flush toxins and bacteria from your bladder; prevent digestive issues; regulate blood pressure and body temperature; protect various organs, tissues, and joints; and regulate sodium or electrolyte balance in your system (Harvard Health Publishing, 2020). I recommend dr̄ half your body weight in ounces per ̄ tad more on super sweaty days.

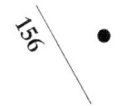

In addition to these techniqʳ that includes eating clean anͺ enhance the body's blood circuͺ help the lymphatic drainage process and the body's ability to expel toxins.

Impact on Blood Pressure

The World Health Organization (WHO) recommends keeping a count on sodium intake because of its effect on blood pressure. As per the WHO's recommendation, reducing sodium intake to less than 2 grams a day, which is almost 5 grams of salt per day, for all adults will prevent hypertension, cardiovascular diseases, coronary heart diseases, and even stroke (World Health Organization, 2012).

An increase in blood pressure can impact your health in many ways. In many cases, it goes back to the point of salt sensitivity. For instance, sodium intake can impact a person's blood pressure but not affect another's at all. Age, weight, and, in many cases, race also play a significant role in salt-sensitivity issues (Cleveland Clinic, 2017).

An increase in blood pressure typically comes with certain signs and warnings. It is critical to comprehend a few symptoms of high blood pressure to prevent any problems. So, here are some symptoms you should be aware of:

- severe headaches
- exhaustion

  vision problems

  difficulty breathing

- irregular heart rhythm
- blood in the urine or nosebleed
- pounding sensation in the chest, ears, and neck

Apart from these signs, some people can get seizures, sweating, nervousness, blood spots in the eyes, sleeping issues, and feelings of confusion as well. Fluctuations in blood pressure can cause serious health issues, so keeping a blood pressure monitor at home or measuring your pressure often is a good idea if you are concerned (Sachdev, 2023).

According to the National Library of Medicine, hypertension can most affect organs such as the kidneys, heart, and brain. These are the target organs that are more likely to be damaged in cases of uncontrolled blood pressure (Mensah et al., 2002).

Let's look at a few ways rising blood pressure or hypertension can damage your health (Mayo Clinic, 2022):

Heart

High blood pressure can lead to several types of cardiovascular issues. Conditions such as an enlarged left heart, coronary artery disease, and even heart failure are very common for people suffering from long-term hypertension. The blood supply to the heart gets affected by the blood pressure because arteries get damaged from the pressure that is applied to supply blood to the heart. Similarly, when the heart pumps very fast to meet the circulation of blood in the body, it causes an enlarged left heart. Moreover, hypertension can cause so much stress on the heart that it fails to work, causing severe health conditions and even death.

Kidneys

Blood vessels and those connected to the kidneys can be damaged because of hypertension. For the kidneys to function and filter waste from the body, it is imperative to have healthy blood vessels. Kidney scarring, also known as glomerulosclerosis, leading to kidney failure, is one of the conditions that a rise in blood pressure can aggravate. In such cases, the blood vessels that connect to and are in the kidneys get so damaged that they start preventing the kidneys from filtering the toxins from the body, which can even lead to kidney failure.

Brain

The body, especially the brain, depends heavily on healthy blood circulation. A dysfunctional blood supply to the brain can lead to a variety of disorders, including transient ischemic attack (TIA), dementia, and stroke. TIA is also referred to as a ministroke. It is caused by high blood pressure due to blood clots and disruption of the supply of blood to the brain. TIA is a small stroke; however, it may also be a sign of a more serious or larger stroke. When the brain is deprived of nutrients and oxygen, the brain cells get depleted. Hypertension can cause ruptures or leaks in the blood vessels, which can further lead to stroke. Apart from these conditions, mild cognitive impairment and dementia are also conditions that can result from prolonged hypertension issues.

Eyes

The blood vessels that connect to the eyes can get damaged due to hypertension. High blood pressure can cause conditions like retinopathy, optic neuropathy, and choroidopathy. Retinopathy can cause the eyes to bleed, blur the vision, and, in many cases, also cause the eyes to lose vision. Choroidopathy is a condition where there is fluid accumulation under the retina, which can cause distorted vision and loss of vision. Optic neuropathy refers to nerve damage that is caused by hypertension; blood circulation gets blocked, which further damages the optic nerve, causing bleeding and loss of vision as well. High blood pressure can also cause other conditions such as glaucoma, retinal vein occlusion, hemorrhages, narrowing of blood vessels, and stroke risk.

High blood pressure is a risk factor for numerous health problems, and it is considered to be extremely risky to have hypertension when pregnant or with an underlying medical condition, like diabetes. From memory to vision, almost every aspect of the body and mind can be harmed if hypertension is not kept in check regularly.

Personal Anecdote

Left turn here and unrelated to blood pressure per se, but health and heart related for sure: One surprising thing I heard recently was about a colleague of my husband. He was boarding a flight and noticed that his legs were unusually fatigued from walking through the airport. He later felt a heaviness in his chest and a pain in his arm. Now, the symptoms of chest pain and arm pain are total red flags we all have heard about, but the heaviness in his legs was new. He listened to his body, left the airport, and headed for the Emergency Room. He had a 70% blockage in the "widow maker," a common vessel to be occluded and cause sudden death. He was able to get a stint put in and lived to tell the tale. He cautioned my husband and their fellow desk jockey colleagues to be aware of that symptom that likely saved his life, so I'm passing it along here too.

Strategies for Managing Sodium Intake

One of my very dear friends would wake up every morning looking like she was three months pregnant. I would wonder how that could be true because I would be with her most of the time, and she was a very light eater. Every morning before heading off to work, she would look at the mirror and, with her tiny fingers, press on her stomach, and it would look and feel swollen. She would lose her confidence for the entire day by starting the day in a bad mood!

This continued for a long time until we thought of investigating what she had been consuming the previous day and what was making her feel like this. We found out that the food she was eating almost every evening, though lower in calories, was pretty high in salt content. She was an ardent lover of soups, so she would use the bouillon powder and soup mixture to prepare her dinner soup, and that was, in fact, causing the extreme bloating every day!

As we know, sodium can be one of the culprits for many of your health conditions. From water retention issues to managing your blood pressure, what you eat and drink plays a significant role. Controlling your salt intake can be a great step toward improving your health.

Here are a few strategies that could help you manage your sodium intake:

Pink Himalayan Salt

According to Healthy Human Life in an article published in Sept 2023, updated October 2023, Pink Himalayan salt has many benefits (*Incredible Benefits of Himalayan Salt*, 2023):

Nutritional Benefits

- For centuries, people who live in "Blue Zones" have relied on a Mediterranean diet. Sea salt is a central part of the Mediterranean way of eating that studies show leads to longevity. Himalayan salt's rich mineral content can help your body detoxify.

- Himalayan salt contains more than 80 minerals and elements, including potassium, iron, and calcium. All of these minerals aid our body's natural detoxification process and promote the removal of bacteria. It contains less sodium than processed table salt and lowers blood pressure. Table salt is highly processed and contains fewer minerals and more sodium than Himalayan salt does. When you swap table salt for Himalayan salt, your body has an easier time processing it because it doesn't require as much water to clear out the excess sodium as it would have if you had consumed table salt.

- To boot, Himalayan salt is naturally rich in iodine, which food companies add artificially to table salt after processing. The natural iodine in Himalayan salt is very effective at helping your body create an electrolyte balance, helping your intestines absorb nutrients, and lowering blood pressure. Contrary to what most people believe, Himalayan salt can aid hydration. Want a great post-workout hack? Drink some Himalayan salt and lemon water.

- The average adult body is approximately 65% water. If we don't drink the 64 ounces or so of water we all need a day (as most of us don't!), our bodies feel it. If the body's water content drops by as little as 2%, we will feel fatigued. How can Himalayan salt and lemon water help? The same way popular sports drinks do. Essentially, when we sweat or work out, we lose minerals or electrolytes. Drinking water with a pinch of mineral-rich Himalayan salt after a workout can help you regain them and, in turn, boost your energy and hydration.

- Himalayan salt's rich mineral content helps balance the body's pH levels. When your pH levels are balanced, your body has better immunity and is better able to process and digest food.

- Do you tend to wake up at 3 a.m.? There's a reason why! This is one of the most common times of night for people to wake up and struggle with sleep, and it can be linked to salt intake. Between 2 a.m. and 4 a.m., biochemical reactions can occur because of high levels of stress hormones that flush through your system and cause sleep disturbances or interrupt your ability to stay asleep. Studies show that low-sodium diets cause blood volume to decrease in the sympathetic nervous system, which, in turn, activates adrenaline and the fight-or-flight response. For a great night's sleep, try mixing some raw honey with a pinch of Himalayan salt and either eat it straight or dissolve it in a cup of tea.

Therapeutic Benefits

- Himalayan salt isn't just for eating! Combine Himalayan salt with coconut oil to exfoliate dry, winter skin, or use a pink Himalayan salt lamp to purify your air.

- Holistic medical practitioners tout Himalayan salt lamps for their ability to purify indoor air, reduce allergies, and improve your overall well-being. Salt is naturally hygroscopic, which means that it attracts water to its surface. The light from the Himalayan lamp causes the water absorbed by it to evaporate quickly. So, although there are few studies on Himalayan salt lamps, it makes sense that they would help with mold reduction and allergies.

- A nightstand set with salt (the lamp kind!) is an easy way to improve your mood and well-being. In addition to purifying the air, the glow of Himalayan salt lamps is a great antithesis to the digital light we often look at just before we go to sleep. A growing body of research shows that exposure to "blue light"—the kind that radiates from our phones, computers, and tablets—actually winds us *up* as we are trying to wind *down*.

- Himalayan salt lamps naturally produce a soft, warm glow that is similar to what a candle or campfire would produce. They're the perfect night-lights for your or your kids' rooms.

- Additionally, Himalayan salt lamps produce a small amount of negative ions—odorless, tasteless molecules found in abundance in natural environments, such as mountains and beaches. Some studies suggest that these ions can boost serotonin and alleviate symptoms of depression.

- You can also get rid of that dry winter skin with a homemade Himalayan salt exfoliator. Himalayan salt makes a great natural exfoliator. Mix the salt crystals with olive oil or coconut oil and use it with a warm washcloth or in a warm bath for smoother, softer skin.

- Salt and mineral baths are a great way to relieve sore or cramped muscles. So, soothe sore muscles with a Himalayan salt bath. Mineral baths make it easy for your body to absorb the magnesium and other trace minerals in the salt, which can fortify bones and connective tissue that may be contributing to soreness.

Challenge!

Tomorrow morning, why not add a pinch of Himalayan salt to your water? Squeeze some lemon in it for added nutrients and bring it with you when you're on the go.

Reading Labels and Making Informed Choices

They may seem small, but the impact of even minor positive changes can have a huge impact on your health. By adopting certain modifications in your lifestyle and habits, you can stay healthy and keep yourself safe from many medical challenges now and in the future.

I get it. Measuring your food and the sodium in it every single day can be a grueling task, especially if you have a hectic schedule. However, in America, people tend to consume much more sodium than the recommended amount. This is one of the reasons why the U.S. Food and Drug Administration (FDA) is leaving no stone unturned in its efforts to curb sodium consumption.

While it may seem tedious, reading nutritional facts labels whenever you buy a food item and making informed choices about what you consume and in what portions can help you manage your health (U.S. Food and Drug Administration, 2021).

To help simplify, here are two things to focus on when you read nutritional facts labels:

1. **Per Serving:** Read the Per Serving quantity and guidelines before consuming the food. For instance, most items have a quantity based on one serving. Make sure to read and understand how much is recommended.

2. **Daily Value:** It's important to understand the proper dosage of any item you consume, especially sodium. Keep a note of the percentage of sodium present and monitor how much you are consuming.

Making healthy choices is key to leading a healthy life, but reading and understanding labels can be tricky. Here are some easy tips to help you understand them, according to the FDA (2020):

- If the label of the food product says "salt or sodium free," then that means it has less than 5 mg of sodium per serving.

- "Very low sodium" means less than 35 mg of sodium per serving.

- "Low sodium" means less than 140 mg of sodium per saving.

- "Reduced sodium" means that the product contains 25% less sodium than in its original version.

- "Light in sodium" or "lightly salted" means that the product contains 50% less sodium than in the original state.

- "No salt added" or "unsalted" means that the product may not necessarily be unsalted. It simply means that no salt was added during the processing of the product.

Reading labels helps, but one of the best methods to keep track of how much sodium you consume regularly is to cook and prepare your own food!

Cooking Tips for Reducing Sodium

Let's look at some easy ways to reduce sodium intake when cooking at home:

- **Read the label:** Always check the nutritional labels of the products you buy. A major amount of sodium you consume regularly is found in packaged food items used for cooking and enhancing flavor. Ensure that you read the correct serving size and the sodium content to be sure of how much to use.

- **Remember: Fresh is best:** Buy fresh food instead of processed and frozen food options. Ensure that you check the label to see if brine water has been added to preserve the meat or other products. Opt for local and seasonal fruits and vegetables so you can prepare your food with items that are less contaminated and not grown with extra chemicals and fertilizers. Many long-preserved items contain coatings of preservatives used to keep them fresh for a long time, which is one of the main reasons to choose seasonal food items. Also, shopping for fresh goods will benefit your local farmers and businesses as well!

- **Put down the salt shaker:** Sprinkling extra salt on food while eating is more of a habit than a need and can be harmful in many ways. Avoid keeping table salt on the dining table or even on the counter to prevent the temptation to add more to your food. While cooking, keep the salt level as low as you can. Even if you are making pickles or salads, try to use as little salt as possible.

- **Shop for fresh veggies:** Avoid using canned and salted vegetables; instead, opt for fresh or frozen vegetables. Canned foods can be misleading because you might choose a tuna sandwich, thinking fish is a healthy option, but the brine and sauce that the tuna is packed in can make it heavy on calories and extremely high in sodium. The more you consume fresh meats, fruits, and vegetables, the healthier eating habits you will cultivate.

- **Wipe it off:** You can try a trick like "unsalting" your snacks. If you have a packet of salted and spiced nuts or seeds, you can always use a napkin to clean off the extra salt. Though we know it is best to not consume excessively salty foods, simple methods like this can come in handy when there are no other options. In fact, snacks are the most common means by which unregulated sodium enters your system. Imagine you are at work and your colleague offers you some salted nuts. Your first response might be to take them and munch on them, but it is very important to be wary of what you consume, regardless of the portion. Try keeping a stash of unsalted nuts at your desk!

- **Wash your food first:** Prior to cooking, make sure to rinse foods, including fruits, vegetables, meat products, nuts, and everything that can be washed. This is great for hygiene, and at the same time, it cleans off any salt on the food products. For example, when you plan to prepare a simple chicken salad, make sure to rinse the chicken thoroughly before cooking. This process of draining the salt water out can be very helpful in reducing any extra sodium content. It may sound like one more pain-in-the-butt step, but the amount of harmful sodium content you save yourself from is worth the effort.

- **Opt for homemade:** Use homemade sauces and dressings for your food and salads. This way, you can reduce almost half the sodium that would be present in prepackaged sauces and dressings. Often, when we dine out and order a vegetable salad, we assume that we are eating very healthy and nothing can go wrong but somehow end up bloated the next day. This happens because most of the salads prepared at restaurants are seasoned with sauces and vinegar that are loaded with sodium and various tastemakers. For example, the fish sauce that is used widely contains a whopping quantity of sodium!

- **Avoid artificial flavors:** Bottled and flavoring packets, like ready-made broth cubes, often contain monosodium glutamate (MSG). This is one of the main reasons why you often feel instantly thirsty after having food with a high sodium content, including MSG. Stick to using fewer artificial flavors to enhance the taste of your food. Always go for natural flavors, like garlic, spices, pepper, citrus juice, and salt-free condiments, while preparing food.

While reducing the sodium content in your food can be a great way to achieve your health goals, consuming healthy and natural foods can be much easier and is also one of the best ways to avoid unnecessary sodium. You might be doing all the relevant crunches and cardio to lose weight, but your tummy simply doesn't show any sign of improvement. Make sure to check how much sodium you have been consuming. You may be surprised to find that the quantity is much more than you think!

The bottom line is that no amount of heavy workouts will give you results if you are not watching your diet and salt intake. Eating organic and non-processed food, coupled with a few hours of physical activity a week, can do wonders for your waistline. Eating more fruits and vegetables can help you achieve a balance in your system and make you feel and look fitter in the long run, too.

A clean, well-rounded diet is not only good for your body but can also do wonders for your mind—another reason why checking what and how much is on your plate before you take that first bite is extremely important. Balanced food choices and proper quantities can make a big difference when multiplied day over day, week over week, and month over month. It all adds up, and consistency is key.

Some Salty Scoop!

Let's be honest, when we think of losing extra inches from our bellies, the first thing that comes to mind is cutting down on calories. But do we ever think about cutting out the salt completely? Not really! But there are a few top models in the glam world who swear by avoiding salt before their photoshoots. As a medical professional, I was flabbergasted by the thought of removing salt completely from the diet, as there could be many harmful health repercussions.

I further delved into this subject and discovered that many models follow something called a "salt depletion diet" a few days before their fashion shoots. I understand that sodium has a huge role in making you look and feel bloated and uncomfortable—along with the many other health issues it can cause, which we've already explored—but the dangers of abstaining from it completely are also a thing.

David Gandy, a male model, shared some of his secrets of preparing for a high-profile photoshoot for Dolce &

Gabbana. He mentioned that he adopted the salt depletion diet because salt caused bloating. Two days before a shoot, he would cut out salt from his diet, and then the day before the shoot, he would dehydrate himself by drinking only one glass of water the whole day and taking a hot water bath at night (NewBeauty Editors, 2017)! The whole point here was to have no water retention issue at the time of the shoot. I am giving this example because I, as a professional, intend to make everyone aware of how dangerous adopting such a diet plan can be. I find it so interesting what some professions/people will go through to achieve (completely unrealistic for the day-to-day gal) beauty standards.

However, I should highlight that while there are potential long-term negative effects of a fully "no salt" diet, this does not contradict the prior discussions in this chapter about limiting excessive salt intake. It is important to realize that neither too little nor too much salt is beneficial to your health. Anything done beyond a limit is dangerous.

Time and again, we are reminded of conventional beauty standards by fashion magazines and videos, which often make us doubt our fitness and appearance. That's another reason why prioritizing your health and mental peace is so, so important. Whether it is for your job or to "impress" someone, no amount of validation is worth your physical and mental health. It is the lifestyle that you choose and the healthy options of food and drink that you incorporate into your life that will help you gain a better perspective on health and fitness. Look better *and* feel better with moderate, healthful consistency.

Being aware of what you consume and in what quantity, understanding the role of sodium in your diet and weight issues, and adopting ways to stay fit and healthy is the best gift you can give yourself. When your mind and body start working in sync, you will notice that you start feeling fitter and fabulous in no time! Don't eliminate salt altogether; instead, use it sparingly and in accordance with your health. To become the best version of yourself and to work toward your flat belly, drink enough water, eat a balanced diet, move your body, and think optimistically.

Chapter 2:

Embracing Healthy Fats

The word "fat" has been made into something scary, hasn't it? Perhaps this is due to the widespread negative image of "fat" that has been propagated for a long time. The problem is the generalization of fats as something harmful, which creates a conflicting attitude toward the consumption of fats and their importance and risk in our diets.

I'm sure we all have been told to stay away from fat by our friends, family, colleagues, and the good old interwebs at times. If we learned anything from the 90s, it is that being on a "low fat" diet caused most of us to have weight problems for the first time. The "low fat" foods often substitute additional ingredients to boost flavor and taste that are far worse for us than if we had just left the naturally occurring fat *in*.

Healthy fats, such as polyunsaturated fats and monounsaturated fats, are required for a flat belly and many body operations. Consequently, a sufficient amount of fats should be included in your normal dietary intake for additional nutrition and its benefits. When we talk about fats, many patients are confused about how fats may be helpful and what various examples of fats exist in both of these categories of fat. Yes, it's understandable that distinguishing between healthy and "bad" fats might be tricky if you don't have the right information, so here you go!

Differentiating Between Good and Bad Fats

Fats can be difficult to understand, and for that reason alone, it is very important to have a clear picture of the differentiating factors between good and bad fats. Your health depends on the type of food you consume regularly, and making healthy food choices and habits can help you keep many diseases, especially cardiovascular disease, at bay.

When it comes to fat—or any type of food—overconsumption can be risky. However, eating the right food can be one of the best things you can do for your health and self-care. Let's learn what good fats and bad fats are so you can easily make healthy choices now and in the future.

How Did Fats Earn a Bad Reputation?

In the homes of older generations, having fat-laden food has been a topic of conversation for a long time. Plates full of bacon and eggs were easier to prepare and delicious to eat at the start of a busy and active day. Due to the high-calorie content, fats were traditionally regarded as one of the best sources of energy. The idea then was to consume tasty fats and stay full longer. It wasn't until researchers conducted several studies that we got the idea that some fats might be "good" and some might be "bad."

In the 1930s, Russian scientist Nikolai Anitchkov found that consumption of high cholesterol by animals could lead to a condition called atherosclerosis. In this condition, plaque accumulates in the arteries, constricting them and elevating the risk of heart disease, increasing the chances of heart attack (University of Minnesota, 2006).

Later, during the 1940s and 1950s, cases of cardiovascular disease decreased, which was credited to the wartime rationing system. So, the widespread notion that rich, high-fat food could be dangerous for the heart became common. Interestingly, researchers examined a group of men with similar characteristics and health conditions by monitoring their blood pressure, serum cholesterol, smoking habits, diet, alcohol consumption, and age. They observed that in about 15 years, deaths among these men were mostly from cardiovascular disease, followed by stroke and cancer. They saw that diverse risk factors, like obesity, high blood cholesterol, and hypertension, could be responsible for heart disease. Additionally, saturated fat in the diet was shown to increase cholesterol and, therefore, increase the risk of heart ailments (Keys et al., 1986).

The bottom line of this study was that not all types of fat posed risks, and not all fats were the same. However, over time, the concept and analysis were likely misrepresented, and the fear of any form of fat quickly spread worldwide. Because of widespread misinformation, it is crucial to dispel any misconceptions, get accurate information about everything you ingest, and understand the distinction between good and bad fats.

Good Fats

There are a whole bunch of fats that are great and do not pose any threat to your heart or overall health. These fats are so good for your health that they can even protect you from several ailments and also help lower your blood cholesterol levels.

Let's talk about the fats that are highly beneficial for your wellness. But note that eating too much of anything may be harmful, and because healthy fats also have a considerable amount of calories and triglycerides, consume them in moderation for the optimal outcome.

Here are some of the "good" fats you should include in your diet:

Unsaturated Fats

Unsaturated fats are healthy fats that are considered to be beneficial for your health. Saturated fats stay solid at room temperature, and unsaturated fats, like oil, stay liquid at the same temperature. This is one of the simplest methods to tell them apart. To avoid any confusion, it is also crucial to note that "trans fat" and "saturated fat" are bad types of fat for your body.

Here are a few of the benefits of unsaturated fats:

- They help provide fuel for the body.
- They help protect the organs of the body.
- They improve the absorption of nutrients in the system.
- They support the healthy growth of cells.
- They help produce vital hormones.
- They boost the level of high-density lipoprotein (HDL), which is also known as "good cholesterol."
- They help lower the risk of cardiovascular diseases.

Two of the most important types of unsaturated fats are monounsaturated and polyunsaturated fats.

Monounsaturated Fats

Monounsaturated fats (monounsaturated fatty acids, or MUFAs) stay liquid at room temperature but can turn semi-solid when kept in a very cold setting. Plant-based oils, like olive oil, canola oil, safflower oil, sesame oil, and canola oil, are some of the types of monounsaturated fats. Seeds, nuts, avocados, and peanut butter are also rich sources of this fat.

This type of fat can not only be helpful for your cells and heart but can also be beneficial for weight loss. According to one study, when 124 obese people were given either a diet high in monounsaturated fats or a diet high in carbs for a year, on average, those who consumed monounsaturated fats lost more weight (Brehm et al., 2008).

Polyunsaturated Fats

Vegetable oils, like soybean, corn, cottonseed, sunflower, and safflower, are a few examples of polyunsaturated fats (polyunsaturated fatty acids, or PUFAs). Margarines, salad dressings, and mayonnaise also contain some of these fats. Polyunsaturated fats are liquid at room temperature and stay liquid even when refrigerated. Two of the most important types of polyunsaturated fats are omega-3 and omega-6 fatty acids. Consuming these fats and replacing saturated fats with them can help lower levels of bad cholesterol and boost levels of good cholesterol.

Among the two, omega-3 fatty acids are considered the best for health.

Omega-3 Fatty Acids

Omega-3s are polyunsaturated fats that are crucial for the body to function. These can be obtained only from diet and other supplements because the body is unable to produce them. They are an important part of the cell membranes, help provide structure and support, and further boost interaction among the cells.

A diet rich in omega-3 fatty acids reduces the risk of heart disease, blood clots, arrhythmia (abnormal heart rhythm), some types of cancer, dementia, Alzheimer's disease, and age-related macular degeneration. It also helps lower the triglyceride and cholesterol levels in the blood. Marine sources—fatty fish like salmon, mackerel, tuna, halibut, sardines, herring, pompano, sea bass, and lake trout—are rich in omega-3s. Also, walnuts, flaxseed, canola oil, soy products, and soybeans contain omega-3s to some extent (Cleveland Clinic, 2019).

Bad Fats

The fats that fall in the "bad" category are the ones you need to watch out for, including saturated fats. Saturated fats are solid at room temperature and are very high in low-density lipoprotein cholesterol (LDL), or bad cholesterol. These fats are also called "solid fats" and are some of the most common fats found in the American diet.

Saturated fats are found largely in animal fats and dairy products. Consumption of excessive saturated fat can increase bad cholesterol levels and raise the risk of high insulin resistance and heart diseases. Beef, poultry, pork, eggs, tropical oils (like palm and coconut), high-fat dairy products, and butter are some of the most common sources of saturated fats.

According to the World Health Organization's guidelines, it is essential to keep track of your fat intake to maintain good health. It is also important to follow the right "macro" count for your body. This is the ratio of carbohydrates, fat, and protein you consume daily. You can find generic amounts online, or we can run a custom calculator for you based on your DNA when you visit www.lifelongmetaboliccenter.com.

Artificial trans fats in processed food were banned by the Food and Drug Administration in 2020 (Wellness & Prevention, 2023). Trans-fatty acids and saturated fats can be replaced by polyunsaturated and monounsaturated fats derived from plant sources. Intake of high artificial trans fats and saturated fats increases the risk of type 2 diabetes and heart disease.

How Healthy Fats Support a Flat Belly

When it comes to losing weight and dropping a few inches, people often turn to reducing their fat intake. As previously said, fat is not the sole enemy. While the bad form can lead to major issues, it may be difficult to believe, but good dietary fats can help you lose weight and get rid of stubborn belly fat!

Monounsaturated fats and omega-3 fatty acids are the real deal and can not only help you stay healthy but can also boost your fat loss journey at the same time. According to a study, the consumption of polyunsaturated fatty acids (PUFAs) raises your resting metabolic rate, which is the calorie consumption needed to live. Additionally, it also increases diet-induced calorie burn, which means that there is a higher and faster rate of calorie breakdown of PUFAs in comparison to saturated fats (News, 2012).

Here are a few interesting ways good fats can help achieve a flat belly (Palinski-Wade, 2016):

Extended Digestion

One of the most common reasons for weight gain is the consumption of more calories than needed for the body to function. Constant snacking due to hunger cravings can lead to a high appetite and result in overeating. Studies show how fats and satiety are related. For instance, healthy and balanced consumption of good fats can affect satiety and can even help in controlling appetite by releasing appetite hormones (Samra, 2010).

Research conducted by UC Irvine pharmacologists found that fatty foods like nuts, olive oil, and avocados help curb hunger by transmitting signals to the brain to prevent excessive eating. This theory is opening new doors in treating obesity and related eating disorders (Irvine, 2008).

Reduces Inflammation

Weight gain is often linked with elevated inflammation in the body, and vice versa. Inflammation is the body's natural defensive system, and prolonged inflammation is associated with serious medical conditions, including obesity. With high levels of inflammation, glucose concentration in the body increases, resulting in excessive fat formation as carbohydrates become harder to digest. As the metabolism slows down, the body's weight tends to creep up. As a result, losing extra pounds can be particularly challenging.

A controlled diet and, more so, an anti-inflammatory diet and a healthy lifestyle are needed to reduce inflammation. A well-balanced diet rich in proteins, fiber, and healthy fats such as olive oil, seafood, nuts, and seeds is advantageous. You can reduce the risk of heart disease and type 2 diabetes by avoiding bad fats, reducing alcohol use, and eating good fats regularly. Additionally, you can efficiently decrease belly fat as your energy increases and metabolism improves with an improved diet and effective lifestyle changes (Drop Bio Health, n.d.).

Reduces Stress Hormones

Prolonged stress and exhaustion could be the reasons behind the production of the stress hormone cortisol in the body. This is a common reason for an increase in fat around the belly and overall weight gain. Good fats, especially omega-3s, can help reduce stress hormones and help cut down extra fat from the body, mainly the belly region, at the same time (Palinski-Wade, 2016).

Incorporating Healthy Fats Into Your Diet

At this point, you are aware of precisely how important it is to include healthy fats in your diet every day to keep both your body and mind in good health. A variety of medical conditions, including those with signs and symptoms that have no known etiology, may have nutrition and food imbalance as their underlying cause. These include a persistent sense of exhaustion or lack of energy; dry skin, hair, and nails; shifts in mood; and, more often than not, weight gain or loss due to prolonged stress and anxiety.

A little planning and discipline are all you need to start a healthy lifestyle. Including good fats in your diet is not that big of a challenge, as most of the food products in that category taste quite good. Nuts, seeds, fatty fish, full-fat yogurt, cheese, and avocados are some splendid choices you can make to include good fats in your diet.

Here are a few ways you can incorporate healthy fats into your regular diet to reap maximum benefits:

- **Check the labels**: Always check the labels of food products to monitor how much fat is in the food you eat. You will be able to consume fat and monitor the quantity with this method.

- **Savor as you eat:** Eat food slowly and make sure to chew thoroughly. This will help in the breakdown of calories and also reduce your appetite by making you feel full, preventing overeating.

- **Monitor your portions:** It's important to control your portions while eating. For example, no matter how hungry you may be, try eating a healthy portion rather than stuffing yourself with excess food. Use a smaller plate to avoid grabbing too large of portions.

- **Stock up on healthy snacks:** Keep some nuts and seeds handy at home or work to snack on whenever you get hungry. This will prevent you from eating something unhealthy when hungry. You can purchase individual serving sizes to prevent overeating larger quantities without realizing it.

Fats are a great source of energy, and when you incorporate healthy fats into your diet, you will start noticing the difference in your health. They not only replenish your body and mind but are also helpful for your weight-loss journey. Knowing and counting your macros can be the best way to reduce belly fat and the heavy feeling in your body. Balance those good fats with an appropriate amount of carbohydrates and protein as well to get the most bang for your buck.

Cooking Techniques for Maximizing Benefits

If you have been wondering how to incorporate healthy fats into your home cooking, here are a few simple ways to create yummy food with great health benefits:

- **Garnish your food with seeds and nuts:** This can be an amazing way to increase nutrients and healthy fats. Sprinkle nuts or seeds over your favorite bowl of oatmeal in the morning or salad during the day. This will not only add a zing and flavor to your food but also benefit your overall health.

- **Use olive oil:** Olive oil is anti-inflammatory and considered to be extremely healthy. Every time you cook, drizzle some olive oil on it. Whether you are cooking sautéed vegetables, preparing pasta, or making some salad dressing, make sure to use olive oil for great health benefits.

- **Try canned fish:** Canned fish is an option for those with busy schedules who are also not very keen on cooking their meals. You can stock your fridge with canned seafood, like tuna and salmon, and use it while preparing food of your choice. Add some tuna to your sandwich and you will get a healthy dose of good fats along with a protein source. Trader Joe's carries canned tuna with zero added sodium.

- **Stock up on avocados:** Avocados are a great source of healthy fats and have many health benefits. Use fresh avocados to make toast, guacamole, or any food item of your choice. If available, try to include avocados in your diet regularly (Ball, 2022).

Planning Ahead

Preplanning is one of the most effective ways to stay on track with your goals. Incorporating healthy fats into your diet is similar, so one of the best methods to manage how much of each kind of food you consume is to prepare and organize your meals ahead of time. If you have your meals prepared, you'll not only take less time to decide what to eat, but you'll also be more mindful of what you put in your mouth.

You can precisely track your calorie intake in this manner, which will be very beneficial for your fitness and weight-loss goals. This is also great for those with busy lifestyles. Preplan according to your macros on Sunday. Shop, chop, and prep foods. Then, Monday through Friday, just eat what you have planned. No thinking is needed during the busy work week!

Watch Your Weight With Fats

It's interesting to think about how fat might help you lose weight and shrink your waistline. In this chapter, I have drawn a clear picture of how there are distinct and different types of fats and that each has its role to play in either harming your health or protecting you from many conditions. How you want to feel can depend on what type of fat you choose to consume!

Fats act as a fuel that helps keep your body going, similar to carbohydrates and proteins. The famous Halle Berry, the 57-year-old actress, has many times shared her experience with trying a high-fat diet to stay fit and prevent diabetes. She is particular about having healthy fats, like avocados, on her plate daily. Similarly, LeBron James, the famous basketball star, also followed a high-fat diet to get his abs more ripped and healthy (Lawler, 2018).

Every person is unique in terms of their health conditions, food sensitivities, and metabolism levels, so it is extremely important to get the right plan for you.

Simple Exercises to Help Burn That Hard-To-Lose Belly Fat

The benefits of a healthy diet with the right amount of good fats are immense. However, when you add a few effective exercises to your routine, your journey from a flab belly to a flat belly can become much easier.

Here are a few workouts that can be super effective in the process:

Cardio or Aerobics

Belly fat, which is visceral fat, is more stubborn than fat in other areas. Doing cardio or aerobic exercise most days can help control your belly fat. Cardio exercises, like running, walking, rowing, swimming, cycling, and jogging, are known to burn a lot of calories, resulting in effective weight loss. However, if you have any underlying health issues, do not pressure yourself into trying difficult exercises.

Make sure to start slow and gradually increase the pace as much as your body can do safely. For those with health conditions, one of the best cardio exercises that never fails is simply walking! So, put those headphones on and take a brisk walk out in the park for a few minutes every single day. Enjoy the warm sunshine and fresh air and take some deep, cleansing breaths.

Weight Training

Weight training is highly beneficial for reducing belly fat. When combined with resistance training, these workouts can boost your metabolism and reduce your body fat. Squats, lunges, tricep kickbacks, and bicep curls are some exercises that show results effectively.

However, make sure to weight train using lighter weights at first, and only then gradually try heavier weights. Lifting weights can improve your metabolism, improve body composition, and burn more calories.

Abdominal Exercises

Like all the other exercises, you should start ab exercises gradually and then increase the intensity. Abdominal crunches, bicycle crunches, planks, and leg lifts are some of the most effective abdominal exercises.

Along with these, the practice of lower abdominal workouts can also be beneficial to boost your strength, posture, balance, and self-confidence. There are a few specific exercises, like mountain climbers, leg raises, scissor kicks, toe touches, and knee tucks, that have also proven to be highly effective in reducing belly fat.

Interval Training and High-Intensity Interval Training (HIIT)

High-intensity interval training, or HIIT, is a combination of intense and varied exercises. For example, during a workout, a very intense and difficult exercise is done for some time and then followed by something light and easy. Rest breaks are taken in between as well. For example, when you do HIIT, you will work on high-intensity movements for half a minute and then rest for another half a minute. This form of exercise is said to be very helpful in reducing belly fat and regulating your overall body weight.

Pulling, pushing, deadlifting, and squatting are some of the exercises that can fall under this category or the weightlifting category. If you do these intensely followed by breaks, they can help you lose a lot of weight. Similarly, exercises like jumping jacks, burpees, high knees, jump squats, and pushups are said to be equally effective in losing belly fat. When you do steady-state cardiovascular exercises, you burn more calories while you are doing the exercise. When you do a HIIT workout, you burn more calories than in the other 23 hours of the day.

Exercising provides innumerable health benefits. From preventing various diseases to increasing your energy, a good workout can give you peace of mind. An added bonus here is the weight and fat loss from the belly. It is natural that when you lose weight, it is quite difficult to lose weight only from a particular section. No, your calorie burners do not work that way and are not selective in cutting off the fat from your body only from the areas that you like (WebMD Contributors, 2023).

By performing "spot exercises" to the core and abdominal region, you give yourself the best chance at affecting that area. If you can fill it with muscle, it looks more tight and toned overall. The combo of proper macros and specific exercises is the best thing you can do for a fast flat belly.

Moreover, to lose weight, you do not have to have access to a fitness club. You can start working on your body right at home. Neither expensive equipment nor expensive diet foods are needed. Stay cautious and watch out for the red flags in the food that you consume. Lots of things that are available in the market are contaminated with artificial add-ons, so finding the right food and place to exercise every day is your best bet.

Eating the simplest of food and from the original sources is very helpful. For example, instead of opting for supplements for fats, nutrients, and vitamins, try to find the simplest and the easiest available natural food. We should eat the way your grandparents did—with maybe a bit less bacon (wink).

So, whether you plan to win a marathon or simply go for a walk in a quiet park, your fitness and holistic health play a major part in making your vision a reality. The bigger your belly gets, the higher your risk of developing unpleasant health conditions in the long run. No age is too late to start with a fitness goal, and regardless of where you are in life, physically or mentally, make sure to realize that it is *you* who you have to take good care of!

Start giving yourself the importance and love you have been giving others all your life. Work on your health goals now, and no matter your age, make sure to move on with a positive outlook. As you progress with this book, you will feel much more sorted and healthy, and in no time, you will be able to work on your mind and body in full swing. Prioritize yourself and embrace all the good things in life, starting with the "good" fats in your diet!

Chapter 3:

Managing Gaseous Foods

We live in a progressive era that, to a great extent, is committed to diversity, inclusiveness, and optimism. Across the globe, there are different types of people with varied skin colors, cultures, body types, health conditions, and even mindsets. Everyone's bodies are not the same, neither are the ways their bodies react to different types of foods and environments. However, one thing that is quite common worldwide is the problem of gaseous foods and the related issues with bloating, which can contribute to severe discomfort.

We all have moments when we do not feel our best, even if we work out regularly and eat clean. There will be days when you wake up feeling bloated, and just when you plan to wear your favorite outfit, it may suddenly feel a tad tight and uncomfortable. Yes, bloating is real and can be extremely problematic at times. We can't deny that there are certain foods and food products that we may be consuming without even realizing that they could be the reason behind those recurring gaseous moments and bloated days!

What Is Gas and Bloating?

Gas and bloating are parts of the very normal process of digestion. Trapped gas can be extremely painful and is also known as gas pain. Though bloating may not be painful, it does generate a feeling of snugness and unease. The feeling of being puffed up, which can be visible as well, can give a blow to your mental and physical state. Burping, belching, and passing gas are some of the most natural processes that help release unnecessary gas from the body.

Digestive issues can be caused by many underlying health conditions. Aerophagia, the excessive swallowing of air, is one condition, but the food you consume can be one of the biggest culprits. That's why it's vital to gain correct information and create a clear understanding of the foods that can cause such issues. By doing so, you can work on reducing the symptoms and find ways to gain permanent relief from the pain and discomfort caused by digestive issues.

Identifying Common Gas-Inducing Foods

One of the first steps to help control gas formation in your stomach is to keep track of what you eat, when you eat, and how much you eat. Once again, food journaling comes into play. Many types of food are gas-inducing.

Your susceptibility to gas and bloating depends on your tolerance level for these foods. If you have been suffering from gas and problems related to it for some time, here are a few things to watch out for:

Cruciferous Vegetables

Vegetables must, without a doubt, be a regular part of a well-rounded diet. There may be times when you're maintaining a healthy diet and limiting your intake of unhealthy items, but despite your efforts, you still experience flatulence troubles. This might imply that you need to keep track of the vegetables you routinely eat. Many vegetables, such as cruciferous vegetables, have a reputation for causing abdominal discomfort and gas.

Brussels sprouts, cabbage, broccoli, cauliflower, asparagus, bok choy, radishes, watercress, arugula, collard greens, and the like are cruciferous vegetables. When consumed, these high-fiber vegetables can be difficult to digest, which is likely to cause gas formation. These vegetables have oligosaccharides, a form of sugar, called raffinose, which is not present in the human system, making it difficult to break down. Some cruciferous vegetables get digested when they enter the small intestine, but when they enter the large intestine, they do not get digested, causing gas to develop.

Additionally, glucosinolates, or chemicals containing sulfur that are found in these vegetables when broken down in the intestine, form hydrogen sulfide and cause a pungent smell like sulfur when gas is passed (Cording, 2018). Though cruciferous vegetables are rich in nutrients and vitamins, we can't overlook the fact that they play a significant part in causing gas and bloating.

Legumes and Beans

Ever wonder why devouring a meal that includes beans and legumes makes your stomach bloated? Well, the beans and legumes are to blame, not you, if you experience just the slightest bit of farting after eating! Fermentable fibers called oligosaccharides are found in beans, similar to those of cruciferous vegetables, which are hard to digest and can cause gas and bloating.

Fiber can cause bloating, flatulence, and stomach pain. Although a high-fiber diet has numerous health advantages, it can also have some negative effects if it is abruptly consumed in large amounts. For example, if you decide to include a large bowl of a certain bean in your diet all of a sudden, then your body will react, causing gas and bloating because it will take time to get used to it. However, if you consume beans frequently, your body may become acclimated to them, and your gas problems may eventually disappear (Cleveland Clinic, 2023).

Studies show that certain beans, like black-eyed peas, pinto beans, and vegetarian baked beans, can cause more flatulence than other beans. Lentils, broad beans, chickpeas, and peas are some of the other food items that cause bloating. The prime reason behind this could be that people have varying tolerance levels for different beans (Winham & Hutchins, 2011).

Bloating and gas issues can be highly uncomfortable and can affect your everyday life. Apart from fiber-rich items, like legumes and beans, some dairy products, whole-grain cereals, some fruits and vegetables, and even chewing gum can add to the problem of indigestion and gas formation. However, it's not advisable to avoid fiber-rich and nutrient-rich foods like these because of their many other health benefits. It is best to go ahead and eat these good-for-you foods, but find a solution to reduce the bloating and gas.

Here are a few ways you can do so:

- **Walk:** Walking can improve blood circulation and bowel movements, making it very effective at reducing gas. Try taking a walk after every meal to reduce flatulence and digestive issues.

- **Practice yoga:** There are numerous yoga poses that can help release gas from the gastrointestinal tract. Child's pose, squats, and happy baby pose can all be very beneficial for releasing gas and minimizing bloating.

- **Try an over-the-counter solution:** Anti-gas pills and medications are available to reduce gas and its effects. Peppermint capsules are also commonly used to relieve gas and bloating. However, medication should be taken only with a medical practitioner's consultation.

- **Utilize essential oils:** The use of certain essential oils, like curcumin and fennel, is effective in reducing bloating and gas. Use them in proportions that are recommended by a professional to avoid any side effects.

- **Relax:** Gentle massage on the abdomen, a warm bath, and other relaxation methods can be very helpful in reducing the symptoms of gas and bloating.

- **Use digestive enzymes:** Having a digestive enzyme like Beano with these foods can help your body digest them with less or even sometimes no gaseous effect.

Additionally, adopting a healthy lifestyle, eating healthy food, and staying hydrated at all times can help reduce bloating problems. For example, taking probiotics, reducing sodium intake, and avoiding only those gas-prone food items for *you* can be great for your overall well-being. Lifelong Metabolic Center offers a fab probiotic if you are interested in beginning to take one on a regular basis.

Although the vast majority might not perceive gas and bloating problems as serious, it's crucial to understand when you should see a medical professional.

Here are a few symptoms that you should watch out for:

- diarrhea
- fever
- vomiting
- appetite loss or gain
- abdominal pain

- weight loss

- blood in stool

Bloating can also be caused by water retention problems that could subside with adequate water intake in a few days. However, if the above symptoms continue for an extended time, then you need to visit your doctor as soon as possible.

Understanding Digestive Processes

The human digestive system consists of the gastrointestinal tract (GI tract), also called the digestive tract, and organs, such as the gallbladder, pancreas, and liver. The digestive tract is also made up of hollow organs comprising the mouth, esophagus, stomach, small intestine, large intestine, and anus.

All of these organs function together to break down the consumed food into nutrients and energy. These nutrients enter the bloodstream and help the cells in the body repair and grow. The food is broken down into different parts, such as carbohydrates, fats, vitamins, and proteins, which have specific functions in the body.

Digestion is highly crucial for the body to operate and stay healthy. For example, it is through the digestive process that proteins are broken down into amino acids, carbohydrates into sugar, and fats into glycerol and fatty acids. So, how does the digestive process work? Let's dive into a few specifics to understand it clearly:

When you consume food, your actions and motions, like chewing, mixing, and squeezing, help break down the food. The digestive juices, enzymes, stomach acid, and bile play a major role in digestion.

Here are examples of how each organ in the digestive system helps in the digestion process:

- **Mouth:** The digestive tract starts with the mouth. The saliva, which is a digestive juice, helps soften the food that you eat and also helps break down the food.

- **Esophagus:** Once the food is chewed in the mouth, the peristalsis helps push the food farther down through the esophagus and into the stomach.

- **Stomach:** The stomach lining has glands that produce enzymes and stomach acid, which play a huge role in breaking down food.

- **Pancreas:** The pancreas produces the enzymes that are responsible for the breakdown of proteins, fats, and carbohydrates. Additionally, it helps deliver the digestive juices to the small intestine through ducts, which are small tubes.

- **Liver:** The liver produces bile and pancreatic juice, which helps in digesting lipids and vitamins. Bile is transported through bile ducts from the liver to the gallbladder and the intestine.

- **Gallbladder:** The gallbladder helps store bile in between food consumption. It also helps squeeze bile through the bile ducts to the stomach while food is being eaten.

- **Small intestine:** The small intestine produces digestive juices that amalgamate with pancreatic juice and bile and helps in the digestion of proteins, fats, and carbohydrates. The microbiome, or the bacteria in the intestine, also further helps in the digestion of carbohydrates.

- **Large intestine:** The bacteria in the large intestine helps digest nutrients and also helps make vitamin K.

- **Anus:** After digestion is completed, waste products become stool and are secreted through the anus, completing the entire digestive process.

The nutrients in the body are mostly absorbed by the small intestine. The circulatory system of the body transfers nutrients to various other parts of the system. Glucose, fatty acids, amino acids, and glycerol are some of the substances that are needed by the body to grow, repair the cells, and get energy (*Your Digestive System & How It Works*, 2023).

How Gas Is Produced in the Digestive Tract

Because there are multiple possible causes of gas formation in the digestive tract, let's explore it in more detail (*Symptoms & Causes of Gas in the Digestive Tract*, n.d.):

- **Swallowed air:** As we already know, when you swallow more air than normal, it can cause gas and gas symptoms. This can be caused by chewing gum, drinking carbonated drinks, eating quickly, smoking, and even wearing loose-fitted dentures.

- **Bacteria in the intestine:** The gut microbiome in your system comprises countless bacteria, fungi, and viruses that play a significant role in digestion. The bacteria in the large intestine helps in the breakdown of carbohydrates. However, food items with high concentrations of starch, fiber, and sugar are difficult to digest, which causes gas formation.

- **Health conditions:** Many preexisting and underlying health conditions can be the reason why gas forms more frequently. Celiac disease, constipation, gastroparesis, gastroesophageal reflux disease, obstruction in the GI tract, lactose intolerance, dietary fructose intolerance, and ovarian, colorectal, or stomach cancer are some of the diseases that are said to cause gas problems.

Though gas problems are more common than w
imagine and not always caused by severe he_
problems, it is always a good idea to consult a doctor _
symptoms like constipation, abdominal pain, weight loss,
or diarrhea persist for a long period of time.

Strategies for Minimizing Gassiness

It is natural to crave foods that cause gas issues, but even the thought of their aftermath can be distressing. However, some of the so-called "gaseous" foods can be prepared in such a way that they do not produce gas when eaten. Though it may sound tedious, with a few tweaks to the food you prepare and other techniques, it is possible.

For example, in many households, legumes are soaked overnight before being cooked the next day. This is done not only to make the legumes softer but to also reduce the compounds in the food that can cause flatulence and indigestion. This is the case for some cruciferous vegetables, too. Cauliflower, for instance, is boiled or steamed, and the water is drained to further cook or just stir-fry it.

Numerous herbs and condiments are known to reduce bloating and gas. For example, probiotics and even herbs with carminative properties, like ginger, rosemary, fennel, sage, oregano, basil, clove, coriander, peppermint, and cumin, can be extremely beneficial in reducing gas issues. By incorporating these herbs and spices while cooking food, you can reduce flatulence and bloating. Similarly, chamomile, caraway, spearmint, parsley, and dill are considered great options for maintaining a healthy gut.

Apart from these natural remedies, sitting up straight during and after eating, taking a walk after a meal, eating frequent but smaller portions, drinking water at room temperature, and eating slowly are some easy ways to curb gas problems. Most of the medication for gas contains activated charcoal, simethicone, and galactosidase, which help in the digestion of food. Some people rely on these medications, and there are others who do not find them effective (Dallas, 2023).

Another interesting way to boost your digestive health is by combining foods! Our food consists mostly of proteins, carbohydrates, and fats. Proteins are digested somewhat slowly, carbohydrates are digested quickly, and fat is digested the slowest of all.

Here are a few points to note about combining foods for improved digestion (Troupe, 2018):

- **Don't mix starch and protein:** Try to avoid starches and protein together if possible. Though it is such a normal and tasty combination, eating a steak with loaded mashed potatoes can aggravate your flatulence problems.

- **Always include veggies:** Try to include vegetables even if you are cooking any form of protein, like meat, fish, cottage cheese, etc. This combination of foods is easy for digestion and lowers gas issues.

- **Eat fruit separately:** Mixing fruits in juice form together or with vegetables may not be a good idea. Consume fruit separately without mixing it with other meals. Ensure to eat melons separately.

- **Rely on good fats:** Healthy fats are great for your health and can be paired with numerous food items.

Observing and understanding your food is very important, and keeping a journal of what food triggered your gas can be beneficial in the long run, too. Avoiding it and calling it natural every time you puff some gas out of your body will not win friends and influence people.

Is Your Weight-Loss Diet Making You Gassy?

I intend to provide genuine information to everyone reading this and support you on your route to fitness using my expertise and experiences collected over the years. I'm sure there are several people who have been giving their heart and soul to reducing weight but are facing the typical hurdle of simply feeling gassy or rather sick every time they eat healthy food. You know that everything on that diet plate is healthy, yet there must be something that is just aggravating the situation and being of no help in the process.

To better grasp the situation, consider the following causes that could be making your diet problematic:

The "Diet" Foods

You enter the supermarket and hit the food section, and the most common site that you see these days is the endless number of aisles, all stocked up with low-calorie, no-fat, and all kinds of "diet foods." In the same context, the number of sugar-free and different sugar substitute options is way too many to confuse a hurried shopper like me! Well, a hidden culprit for your gas troubles could be found among those highly advertised and modified foods.

For example, if you are trying to reduce your sugar intake and opting for many of these sugar substitute items, then the gas you are experiencing may be because of your intolerance to sugar alcohols, which are also called polyols. They contain fewer calories than normal sugar and are used generously in sugar-free items, like bars and crackers, diet soda, and even yogurt. They can be found in numerous diet food items, and when you overconsume these items assuming they are healthy and not harmful, you often end up feeling sick.

These low-calorie sweeteners are not easily digested because they cause bloating, gas formation, and many other digestive issues, including diarrhea. There are a few fruits and vegetables that are said to contain sugar alcohols, and they, too, can cause gas and bloating. Some of the fruits and vegetables that contain natural sugar alcohols are apples, sweet potatoes, mushrooms, pears, and plums.

So, if you have been facing a challenge to lose weight because your weight issues are making you uncomfortable and sick most of the time, you can do the following:

- **Limit artificial sweeteners**: If you are used to having artificial sweeteners and sugar alcohols, then make an effort to eliminate your intake.

- **Look for hidden ingredients:** Check the labels of all the diet-friendly foods that you intend to consume, as there could be hidden calories, preservatives, and excessive sodium that could worsen your weight issues.

- **Avoid problem foods:** Check for all the items mentioned before in this section and avoid having those in your regular diet.

- **Rely on natural sweeteners:** Use natural sweeteners like honey or small amounts of good old-fashioned real sugar.

Always remember, anything eaten in moderation should be fine. So, instead of buying "diet foods," eat more home-cooked, naturally occurring food or organic options but with portion control (Plowe, 2022).

Fiber

This might sound out of place in this list, but it is a fact that too much fiber in your diet can become a bit difficult to digest. It is always advised to have fiber-rich food when on a weight-loss plan. It helps you stay satiated for a long period and is also nutritious. For example, kidney beans, when eaten in the morning, can make you feel full the rest of the day, which helps reduce your intake of unnecessary calories.

Fruits and vegetables, like pears, strawberries, blueberries, blackberries, oats, carrots, beets, broccoli, chia seeds, bananas, dark chocolates, and cruciferous vegetables, are some of the most common fiber-rich foods you can have while on a diet or to maintain a healthy lifestyle.

So, the dilemma remains: We know how healthy fiber-rich foods are and how often it is advised to have them while trying to lose weight, but how can they be causing extra weight gain and preventing you from reducing those belly inches?

Though the USDA advises including around 25 to 30 grams of fiber in your diet daily, many people often fail to consume the amount of fiber their bodies need. Most of us often run with a fiber-deficit condition without even realizing it. In this situation, when you enter a diet routine and start consciously adding more fiber to your diet, that can lead to more probable weight gain than weight loss.

No doubt, fiber is good for your health, but when consumed in the wrong way, it can create a few problems, like the one mentioned above. Refrain from adding fiber all of a sudden to your diet; rather, do it more gradually. Your body has to adjust to the way fiber-rich food gets added to your system. By understanding this concept of introducing fiber to your system, you will be able to make more effective diet plans and see the best results out of them (Plowe, 2022).

Carbonated Drinks and Juices

Carbonated drinks, like soft drinks, energy drinks, and juices, can be extremely tempting to quench your thirst. Time and again, the importance of drinking adequate water is laid out by experts and medical practitioners. From flushing out waste and toxins from the body and maintaining a normal body temperature to lubricating the joints and keeping you hydrated at all times, the benefits of water cannot be overstated.

Dietitians recommend drinking plenty of water while on a weight-loss plan. However, it has become more of a trend to juice and call it "healthy." It is better to have the full fruit than a blended version of it. Because of this, nutritionists often advise their patients and clients to refrain from drinking juice.

Though advised not to, one of the main reasons why people get tempted to drink carbonated drinks in place of water is because water can get bland and is tasteless. On the other hand, juice, soft drinks, and soda tend to quench your thirst and reduce cravings. If you are a fan of juicing, try to use the complete fruit. The skin of an apple plus the "guts" create a perfect blend of fiber/juice for great digestion and a slower "burn."

Every sip of a carbonated beverage taken through a straw doubles the likelihood of flatulence. This happens because the air bubbles in the drinks are taken in, allowing more air to enter the mouth and cause gas issues. The only way to reduce the ill effects of carbonated drinks is to refrain from them. Instead, you can opt for flavored water with fruits and herbs. Make sure to have unsweetened drinks because it is the hidden calories in foods and drinks that often go unnoticed and contribute to more weight gain and water retention problems.

Working out and controlling your diet will be much easier with a healthy body and mind. Once your bloating and gas formation is treated, it will be much easier for you to focus on losing weight, feeling more confident, and getting much healthier in the long term (Plowe, 2022).

More on Raffinose

Raffinose is an oligosaccharide, a tiny sugar molecule that is found in many vegetables, like Brussels sprouts, beans, broccoli, cabbage, and even whole grains. It is composed of complex carbohydrates, and it also has fructose, glucose, and galactose, all different sugar molecules. Since it is found in some of the most nutritious food sources, it cannot be said that it is bad; it is only when consumed more than needed that it can have side effects like upset stomach, digestion problems, and gas issues.

If you notice that some of the foods containing raffinose are impacting your weight-loss efforts and causing digestion issues as well, you can slow down the consumption of these foods. Instead of completely cutting off these food sources from your diet, you can gradually introduce them and slowly increase the quantity so your body does not react to a sudden change (Plowe, 2022).

Being aware of what you consume and in what portion can be beneficial in your weight-loss journey as well. More often than not, when you are on a journey of weight loss and reducing some weight off the abdomen, being sure of what you eat and what foods can create chaos in your system is very important. As we've seen, there are foods that fall into the category of gassy foods, which can make you feel heavier, bloated, and down. Identifying the foods that trigger your body and brain can help you sail toward achieving your fitness goals.

Regardless of whether you want to prevent or cure a certain illness or lose weight in general, making an effort to understand your body and its response to various types of food and situations is the best approach that you can take in your self-care journey. So, whether you want to lose some belly fat or stop those embarrassing flatulence episodes every now and then, paying attention to the food you consume regularly can be a life-changing experience altogether. By tracking these foods, you can keep in all of the healthy choices that work well with your body and reduce those that cause bloating for you—all working toward your flat belly.

Chapter 4:

Food Allergies and Sensitivities

Doesn't everybody know that one kid who is allergic to *everything*?! You can't have PB and J at the lunch table because Adam might sit there next period. One food might be perfectly fine for one person and cause a horrific reaction in another. Therefore, it's necessary to recognize the difference between food sensitivities and allergies.

Recognizing Allergic Reactions and Sensitivities

When it comes to food allergies and food sensitivities, both conditions are the immune system's response to some of the foods we consume. Though both conditions appear to be similar, they can be completely different with regard to their symptoms.

Food Allergy

Allergic reactions to food include symptoms like itching, rashes, anaphylaxis, dizziness, swelling, and hives. Food allergies are caused by a response of the immune system and can be dangerous at times. Some of the most common foods that can cause allergies are eggs, soy, milk, shellfish, nuts, and wheat. The allergy can appear within a short period of time, and immediate medical help is required for severe symptoms.

For instance, I recall a day when all of my friends and I were enjoying a small picnic near the lake in the city. Music and laughter filled the air, but none of us imagined that the relatively simple dish we were eating could be so hazardous or that Raul, a friend of ours, would take a mouthful of it without knowing what was coming. It was a basic sauce with a few ground peanuts in it, and it turned out that Raul was allergic to peanuts. We were aware that he was allergic, but we had no idea that the sauce contained a peanut combination. Without wasting any time, we called for help and managed to take him to the emergency room on time! That was one of the scariest instances that I've come across to date.

Signs and Symptoms of Food Allergy

Serena Williams, the world-renowned American professional tennis star, and Brian Matusz, an American professional baseball pitcher, are both allergic to peanuts! Steve Martin, the famous American actor, writer, musician, and comedian, is allergic to shellfish, and Bill Clinton, the 42nd president of the United States, is said to be allergic to flour and chocolate! (Nohe, 2020). Food allergies can be clingy, quite difficult to get rid of without proper medication and care, and can happen to almost anyone. If not recognized and taken care of at the right time, they can lead to serious problems.

Countless people are allergic to one thing or another. However, serious food allergies can be lethal, so having a clear understanding of the allergens that affect you and the people around you can be of great help during emergencies.

Here are a few common signs and symptoms of a food allergy:

- having a tingling sensation and itching in the mouth
- sudden development of hives, rashes, and even eczema
- swelling of the lips, mouth, tongue, face, throat, and other parts of the body
- nasal congestion, breathing difficulty, wheezing conditions
- unexplained abdominal pain, nausea, diarrhea, and vomiting
- change in voice and difficulty swallowing food
- lightheadedness, dizziness, and even passing out or fainting

- a sudden drop in blood pressure, palpitation, and rapid pulse

The symptoms of a food allergy can vary; sometimes, they can last for just a few minutes, and at other times, they can last for a few hours. Symptoms like swelling of the tongue can be extremely dangerous, as it can cause obstruction and tighten the airways for breathing. In many cases, a few signs are so mild that people often do not realize that they are getting an allergic reaction. However, in some cases, the signs may be strong and can cause a person to weaken and lose consciousness in a matter of a few minutes (*Food Allergy*, 2021).

Visit a Doctor

If you notice even a slight allergic reaction, it is best to visit a doctor to understand the condition. Watch out for triggers every time you eat something that makes you feel uncomfortable. Most importantly, if you have signs, especially shortness of breath, constriction of airways, and rapid drop of blood pressure, then you must immediately rush to the nearest emergency room.

Diagnosis of Food Allergy

There are a few points the doctor will investigate when diagnosing a food allergy. In addition to going over your detailed medical history and your family's allergy history, here are a few questions they might ask:

- How long does it take for your allergy symptoms to develop?

- What food are you sensitive or allergic to?

- What are the primary signs that you experience when you have an allergic reaction?

These are some of the most common queries that almost every medical professional will make to understand your situation. However, as a responsible individual, you can keep track of which medications or foods you know you are allergic to and ensure that you provide accurate information to your doctor.

Tests for Food Allergies

Tests and examinations for food allergies are typically skin and blood tests. Medical professionals perform these tests to get a clear analysis of your specific allergies. Also, if you want to know what food is giving you allergies, then there are allergy testing methods that can help you understand your condition.

An allergist or medical professional will ask you various questions like the ones mentioned above about your allergies. This is one of the ways they will recognize what food items are giving you allergic reactions. However, simply performing an allergy test will not solve your problems. It takes dedication and effort on your end as well to prevent and work on your food allergy issues.

Here are the three most common tests that medical professionals conduct while figuring out food allergy conditions:

- **Skin test:** This is considered to be the quickest way to figure out food allergies. A drop of liquid is placed on the skin, and it is pricked with a needle. After waiting for some time, the doctor will observe any reaction, like the formation of a small bump or redness, to be sure of an allergic reaction. If the red bump resembles a mosquito bite, then that can indicate that you are allergic to the food. In the same test, if your skin does not react in any way, then that indicates you are not allergic to the food. This food allergy test can be performed on several food items.

- **Blood test:** It is a method used to find out about food allergies. A medical professional will take some blood and then be exposed to various allergens. The test sample is taken to the laboratory, and the result is awaited. Most doctors do not encourage this way of testing for allergies because it takes almost a week to get the reports back from the laboratories. However, it is said that tests like this and even the skin test are not completely foolproof and can have different results.

- **Controlled food challenge:** This is a test that is not used by doctors often. It is said to be harmful to people with chronic allergies. This is done in rare cases where the doctor gives a few samples and waits for any reaction to pinpoint the exact food that is causing the food allergies. It is because of this procedure that this method is considered to be unsafe and risky. However, you should opt for this option only when you are physically present in a medical facility where, even if something goes haywire, it can be controlled by experts (WebMD Editorial Contributors, 2022).

To find a solution to a problem, it is always a good idea to acknowledge the existence of a problem first. In the same way, your allergies can be handled and taken care of only when you recognize the main factor that is the root cause. Correct diagnosis and proper tests are of utmost importance.

Food Sensitivity

Food sensitivity, also called food intolerance, includes symptoms like gas, bloating, constipation, diarrhea, nausea, and cramps. Food intolerance is not caused by an immune response but by the body's inability to digest a certain type of food. Additionally, it is not a life-threatening condition. It is more like feeling gassy after having a bite of cheese or getting a severe toothache after having something sweet.

Food is a necessity, and staying away from various types of food can be impossible. There may be many times when we eat something for the first time without realizing we are sensitive to it. So, being cautious of what we eat and observing what foods cause sensitivity and allergy issues is vital. There are many tests that can check the causes of different allergies and sensitivities and treatments for them as well.

Effects of Untreated Allergies on Digestive Health

Allergies can be more than just painful; they can be highly irritating and also impact your regular life. From severe rashes and teary eyes to swollen faces or life-threatening reactions, one small negligence in what you eat can leave you bedridden for a long time. Consider a situation where you are allergic to pollen, but you can't avoid passing through the park or ignoring someone handing you a bouquet of flowers. You can imagine the scenario after that: messy, sickening, and frustrating! Well, in this case, the histamine causes this chaos. However, when it comes to food, it can be extra tricky to understand what is causing an allergic reaction, especially if you've never had one before.

Allergies can adversely affect the digestive system. Food allergies are linked to the gastrointestinal system because the first organ that the food you consume enters is the gastrointestinal tract. Many allergic reactions to the wrong food cause symptoms like abdominal pain, vomiting, and diarrhea. Also, when adopting a healthy lifestyle and losing weight, you often tend to try new types of dietary foods and supplements. Make note of any food that gives you even a slight sign of an allergy, especially when consuming it for the first time.

Studies show that more than 170 food items cause food allergies (*Food Allergy Versus Food Intolerance*, 2019). If undiagnosed and untreated, allergies can affect your digestive health, as around 70% of the immune system is present in the human gut (*Do Allergies Affect Your Gastro Health?* 2023). This makes it highly possible that the cause of your excessive bloating and gas formation could be allergies.

Inflammation and Digestive Discomfort

Inflammation in the gastrointestinal tract could be one of the biggest reasons for digestive discomfort and abdominal bloat. It is one of the primary aspects of the body's immune response. Depending on the duration, symptoms, and level of pain, inflammation can be called either chronic or acute inflammation. Irritable bowel disease (IBD), irritable bowel syndrome (IBS), gastroenteritis, gastroesophageal reflux disease (GERD), along with many other conditions that cause heat, pain, swelling, etc., are some of the inflammation that affects the digestive system.

No doubt, several health conditions are associated with inflammation in the digestive tract, causing discomfort and pain. Crohn's disease and ulcerative colitis are two of the most common health issues connected with IBD:

- Crohn's disease causes inflammation in the digestive tract, and it can affect the areas starting from the mouth to the anus. Pain in the abdomen, fever, loss of appetite, fatigue, weight loss, uneasy bowel movements, and watery and bloody diarrhea are some of its symptoms.

- Ulcerative colitis is an inflammatory bowel disease that begins in the rectum region and moves upward to the colon area. This condition is limited only to the rectum and colon. Diarrhea, discomfort, abdominal pain, and rectal bleeding are some of its symptoms.

Inflammation in any region can be a painful experience, and if the inflammation in the GI tract is not taken care of, then prolonged issues can even lead to the risk of bowel cancer.

Additionally, here are a few more conditions that can add to the problem of inflammation:

Irritable Bowel Syndrome (IBS)

Irritable bowel syndrome is a condition that affects the digestive tract, and many people get severe symptoms. It is a common issue and has to be taken care of medically. Symptoms of IBS are abdominal pain, cramps, bloating, diarrhea, gas, constipation, changes, and irregularity in bowel movement.

The primary causes of IBS are not limited to a single factor. It could be caused due to the following reasons:

- **Infection:** Excessive growth of bacteria can cause bouts of diarrhea and related infections in the intestines. This condition, called gastroenteritis, can be one of the main reasons for IBS problems.

- **Muscle contraction:** The muscles that line the intestine walls contract as the food passes through them. This is a normal digestive process, but if the contraction lasts longer and gets stronger, then various issues, like diarrhea, bloating, and gas, can be the result. On the contrary, if the contraction of the muscles gets slower than normal, then constipation and dry and hard stool can cause severe discomfort and problems.

- **Nerve issues:** The nervous system plays a significant role in the functioning of the digestive system by transmitting signals. However, when the transfer of signals weakens and the connection between the intestine and the brain gets disrupted or very slow, it can adversely affect the digestive process. Some of the symptoms caused by such factors are stomach aches, constipation, and even diarrhea.

- **Stress:** People with high stress levels from an early age are said to experience IBS symptoms more frequently.

- **Gut changes:** Changes in the gut microbiome with alterations in the level and type of bacteria, fungi, and viruses present in the intestine have an impact on the overall health of a person. It has been found that people with IBS have slightly different microbes than those without the condition.

It is vital to consult with your doctor if you experience excessive weight loss, night diarrhea, anemia or iron deficiency, rectal bleeding, or vomiting and if the pain does not subside even after taking over-the-counter medications. Depending on the severity of the condition, your doctor can give you medication or counseling treatments. The good news is that the risk of developing colorectal cancer and alteration in bowel tissue is minimal in this condition (*Irritable Bowel Syndrome*, n.d.).

Gastroesophageal Reflux Disease (GERD)

Gastroesophageal reflux disease is a condition caused by consistent stomach acid that moves back into the tube that connects your mouth and stomach. With GERD, there are moments when you eat something, and after a while, instead of getting a regular burp, you feel the acid from your stomach rise up through your digestive pipe and reach your mouth. This condition is often referred to as acid reflux and can be taxing to your esophagus.

Acid reflux is a normal and common condition most people experience. It can happen mostly after consuming rich, oily, and spicy food. However, if acid reflux gets too frequent, it becomes GERD, which can be controlled by simple lifestyle changes and medications.

Here are a few symptoms to watch out for:

- regurgitation or backwash of food or bitter liquid from the pipes of the intestine to the mouth
- uneasiness and a burning sensation like heartburn in the chest, mostly after eating something
- chest and upper abdominal pain
- dysphagia, the condition of difficulty swallowing
- a feeling of something stuck in the throat

Asthma disorders can also develop as a result of acid reflux at night, which can cause a persistent cough, laryngitis (pain/strain in the voice cords), and other respiratory problems. If any of these symptoms persist for a prolonged period, you should visit your doctor (*Gastroesophageal Reflux Disease (GERD)*, 2023).

Infectious Gastroenteritis

This condition is also referred to as the stomach flu. The inflammation in the stomach and the intestine is caused by bacteria, which further causes vomiting and diarrhea. Some of the most common symptoms of gastroenteritis are stomach aches, watery diarrhea, fever, nausea, cramping, and headache. This condition can also cause mild to severe dehydration, which can lead to lightheadedness, extreme thirst, and dry skin and mouth.

Gastroenteritis is infectious, as it can spread from someone suffering from the condition due to the virus, contaminated water and food, unhygienic conditions, changing diapers, unwashed hands, etc. Rotavirus and norovirus are the two most common types of the virus responsible for the condition. Though very rare, there are some parasites that can also cause gastroenteritis. Swimming in public pools and drinking contaminated water can be huge risk factors for parasites.

There are a few not very common but probable ways to get infectious gastroenteritis, like through the toxins present in certain seafood; excessive consumption of acidic foods; like tomatoes and citrus; metals present in drinking water; and various medications, like antibiotics, laxatives, antacids, and even chemotherapy drugs.

Drinking lots of fluids and gradually hydrating can be helpful. As symptoms like vomiting and diarrhea start subsiding, healthy eating is very important. Avoiding alcohol, dairy, and caffeine is important as well. However, if the symptoms persist and you face severe fatigue and weakness, you should consult with your doctor (DiLonardo, 2018).

Leaky Gut Syndrome (LGS)

Leaky gut syndrome is more of a hypothetical condition, and some doctors do not recognize LGS as a disease that is diagnosed. In this intestinal condition, bacteria, toxins, and food particles go past the intestinal lining into the bloodstream, which can lead to the weakening of the permeability of the intestinal walls, imbalance in the gut flora or microbiome, and further cause several diseases like Crohn's.

Some of the symptoms associated with this condition are constipation, acute diarrhea, bloating, fatigue, headaches, lack of focus, joint pain, skin issues, and inflammation in general. No certain cause for LGS can be pinpointed, though there are certain conditions that could increase its risks, like excessive alcohol consumption, poor nutrition, autoimmune disorders, infections, diabetes, and even consistent stress (Eske, 2023).

Stress

Perhaps "stress" is one of the most frequently used words in our everyday lives. It could be caused by many reasons—physical, mental, environmental, and so on.

Stress can have adverse effects on your gut health, too! Stress can be short term or long term and become chronic depending on the situation and condition. If you are facing short- or long-term stress, some of the signs you might experience are loss of appetite, gastrointestinal issues like indigestion, and stomach aches. Chronic stress can also lead to irritable bowel syndrome and many other serious GI conditions.

Maintaining a healthy diet, including prebiotics and probiotics, can help increase the good bacteria present in the gut and help ease the digestive process (Hill, 2018).

Altered Gut Bacteria

The human gut is said to contain more than 100 million microbes, comprising bacteria that are good for overall health. These good bacteria help fight the bad bacteria that can cause severe health risks and conditions. According to Dr. Friedman, if there is an alteration or imbalance in the gut bacteria and the microbiome, that can lead to several health issues, including inflammation (Godman, 2021).

Studies show that intestinal microflora plays a significant role in transmitting messages between the brain and the gut, supplying nutrients, helping in cellulose digestion, and synthesizing vitamin K. Because of this, the human microbiome is also referred to as the "second brain," and any imbalance or alteration in it caused by the use of antibiotics, stress, aging, bad dietary choices, an unhealthy lifestyle, or illnesses can lead to several conditions, including Alzheimer's disease (Dicks, 2022).

Apart from the mentioned conditions, there are a few other areas of concern that could be responsible for aggravating the risk of inflammation and diseases related to digestive disorders. For example:

- **Medications:** Medications used to curb and treat many illnesses, like anti-inflammatory medicines, antibiotics, and even oral contraceptive pills, can cause the risk of conditions like IBD.

- **Genetics:** Genetics can be blamed for increasing the risk of developing many health issues, including inflammatory bowel diseases. Due to cases of gene mutation, the immune system of the human body can be altered to a great extent and further cause issues.

- **Lifestyle and diet:** Lifestyle and diet can be huge factors influencing your health. Consistent consumption of red meat, highly processed food, saturated fat, smoking, drinking alcohol, and a life without much physical activity can lead to the risk of many health complications, such as digestive disorders, inflammation, weight gain, and even conditions of IBD (Godman, 2021).

The importance of microbes in your gut cannot be overlooked. From digesting food to improving your immunity and overall health, microbes can protect you from countless diseases. As we have already seen, an imbalance and alteration in the gut microflora can cause severe health conditions and even weight gain. We cannot ignore that there are numerous advantages of having a healthy gut microbiome to overall gut, heart, and brain health.

Navigating a Flat Belly With Food Sensitivities

A healthy lifestyle with a weight that is on par with your body mass index (BMI), body fat percentage, and muscle mass amounts can be a great feeling overall. Nonetheless, shedding a few pounds and losing a few inches around the belly can be difficult to achieve without a healthy diet and physical routine. And for those who have food allergies and food intolerance, finding the perfect diet can be quite a difficult task.

Of course, to make things easier, there are countless products available on the market that sell with "allergen-free" labels on them. These can be more convenient but can be very costly in the long run. So, why not get a few ideas that can not only help you with your weight loss journey but also help you understand how to keep a distance from foods that can make you sick?

Identifying Alternative Options and Substitutions

Maintaining a weight-reduction regimen can be complicated for those with particular food sensitivities and allergies because many of the foods advised for weight management may not be the best choice for you. The best course of action in this situation is to adhere to a few rules when choosing your meals, along with searching for alternatives and substitutions as much as you can.

Here are a few suggestions:

Consult a Nutritionist

For someone who has allergies or is prone to food intolerance, the first step is to consult with a professional dietician or a nutritionist. In today's world, there is a lot of information given on the internet regarding health conditions, which can cause more damage if false. So, having professional guidance is the best way to understand your allergies and learn methods to keep your condition in check. On the Lifelong Metabolic Center program, we utilize all-natural, anti-inflammatory, and low glycemic foods all outside of the top five food sensitivity groups. In Phase 4, we can do a "reverse elimination" process to determine potential food sensitivities before returning anything to your regular daily intake. We believe it is best to do a metabolic reset utilizing these foods and then help you find the right foods for *you* lifelong.

Keep a Food Journal

One of the most effective ways to keep yourself healthy and in good shape is to be mindful of your food choices. Taking note of the foods that tend to make you feel sick or queasy might not only help you remember the specifics but can also be extremely helpful in an emergency. Making sure to inform the chef or the restaurant staff of any ingredients or food components that you cannot have on your plate is a must every single time you eat out. However, if you feel self-conscious about it, then you can simply ask for the ingredients that have been used in your food. Staying vigilant as well as averting complications before they develop is always better than seeking a solution afterward.

Go for Food Allergy Alternatives

Some of the most common food allergens are milk, eggs, peanuts, tree nuts, shellfish, fish, and soybeans. Though these food items may not be completely replaceable in certain dishes, there are a few other alternatives you can use to still enjoy tastes similar to these.

Here are some of the most widely used food alternatives that people with food intolerance and allergy issues can opt for:

Milk Substitutes

Coconut, soy, oats, almonds, cashews, hazelnuts, rice, potato, sunflower, and macadamia milk can be used to replace cow's milk for a variety of uses. These kinds of milk are created from plant sources and are also rich in vitamins A and D. Studies show that around 80% of milk intolerance cases increase within a span of two to three years. Milk is very commonly used all around the globe.

From milk tea to puddings, there are numerous delicacies that are prepared with it (Solinas et al., 2010).

The risk of lactose intolerance highly persists for people who have food intolerance issues. In most cases, doctors advise people to avoid dairy and milk products completely, and that can be a big challenge for those who crave milk products. In such a case, milk substitutes can be a real win.

Egg Substitutes

Eggs can be a part of countless delicious dishes and are used almost everywhere in the world. They are used in batters, baking, salads, and a wide range of manufactured products as well. This can make it difficult for someone with an egg allergy to find food products without eggs. There could be chances of cross-contamination in many foods, especially while eating out in a restaurant, making it all the more difficult for allergic patients.

Eggs are widely used as binding agents when frying, baking, or cooking food. If you can't use eggs due to allergy, you can use other forms of binding substitutes while preparing your desired dish. For binding, you can use apple sauce, mashed bananas, and ground flaxseed mixed with water. Similarly, gelatin and sometimes corn flour can also be used in place of eggs for cooking purposes.

Wheat Substitutes

Wheat is one of the most common ingredients used for cooking in nearly every part of the world, but many people are also allergic to wheat. Wheat is found in a large number of food products, and it is very difficult to track whether food has been contaminated by wheat.

Celiac disease is distinct from a wheat allergy, despite seeming similar. Wheat allergy has to do with antibodies, but celiac disease is about a reaction to gluten, a type of protein present in wheat that causes immune system problems (Cianferoni, 2016).

There is a wide range of flours available on the market that are gluten and wheat free. Flours made from coconut, almond, oats, and rice are some of the most common substitutes for wheat. These flours are not only helpful in avoiding allergies and sensitivity to gluten and wheat but are also rich in nutritional value, including fiber and minerals. Almond flour, for instance, is known to help control cholesterol issues and can be used just like wheat for baking and cooking. From packaged food that is gluten free to bread and pasta that are made from buckwheat, millet, potatoes, rice, tapioca, and chickpea flour, these are some great substitutes for wheat that you can use to prepare your food.

Protein

There are many cases where people suffer from dietary protein intolerance. This is a clinical syndrome caused by the absorption of proteins through permeable mucosa in the small intestine. It is the protein in cow's milk that causes numerous children to become intolerant of it (Walker-Smith, 1988).

Protein is very important for building muscles, neurological functions, hormonal balance, and overall health. Fish and shellfish are good sources of omega-3 fatty acids and proteins, but people sensitive to and allergic to their proteins have problems consuming them. However, protein is a must in your diet, and if you cannot consume fish or seafood, you can opt for various other protein substitutes, like eggs, yogurt, grass-fed meat, and poultry. Similarly, if you choose a vegetarian diet, then plant-based proteins, like black beans, natto, and lentils, are some great options. Walnuts, chia seeds, and flaxseed are also sources of fiber, minerals, vitamins, and protein (Ruggeri, 2016).

While on a fitness journey, the food you eat does not have to be bland and taste bad. If you are allergic to animal protein, there are many plant-based protein options on the market that not only help you prepare the type of meal you want but also taste just the same! Alternatives and substitutes are always there to help you with your fitness goals and enhance your taste bud experience.

Challenges to Lose Weight With Food Allergies and Intolerance

Checking the scales every now and then can be demotivating if you do not see the result you aimed for. Belly fat is so stubborn that it takes a lot of diet control, exercise, and, most importantly, reduced stress. While these criteria may seem achievable, one thing that remains of primary concern is whether your food allergies and sensitivities are causing hurdles in the process of your weight loss.

Food is an essential part of our lives, and when it comes to health, your diet and lifestyle play a huge role. Weight loss is not just about eating less; it is about eating right. There is no doubt that counting macros is one of the best ways to shed extra weight. It is understandable that allergies and food sensitivity can cause immense discomfort and hurdles in regular life and in your efforts to work on your fitness, but that should not stop you from trying.

Tennis player Novak Djokovic, for example, is known to be gluten intolerant. Interestingly, he grew up in a household that had a pizza restaurant, which meant he was surrounded by bread, pasta, and everything gluten. It wasn't until he entirely eliminated gluten from his diet that his asthma, colds, flu, and allergies disappeared. His family was worried because he started to lose weight and lost around 11 pounds after he ditched gluten. He could, however, sense the good flow of energy and increasing stamina, and rightfully so. A few years later, he won 10 titles, 43 straight matches, three grand slams, and many more (*Is a Food Intolerance Making Weight Loss Difficult?* 2014).

This shows how determination and willpower, even amidst the biggest of temptations, can help you achieve your goals. In Novak Djokovic's case, we can see that staying in an environment with gluten around and staying away from it must have been extremely difficult. Similarly, if we try to understand our health conditions and food intolerances, we will be able to find ways to make tweaks to our diet and lifestyle and work toward achieving our goal of losing weight and some waistline inches, too!

Food Allergy and Weight Gain Connection

How can being allergic to eggs and unable to eat them lead you to gain weight? That does seem bizarre! It is true that food sensitivities and allergies have some link when it comes to the problems of losing weight.

Here are a few ways your food allergies can create some hurdles in your effort to lose weight:

Diet

When you are allergic to certain foods, like eggs, peanuts, and certain fruits, your diet becomes restricted to a few other items only. When on a weight-loss plan, having nutritious and healthy food is very important. However, with food restrictions due to allergies, numerous nutritious foods get eliminated from your regular diet. For example, by cutting eggs, milk, and peanuts from your diet, you reduce the intake of all the goodness that foods like these provide in terms of protein and nutrients. This increases the risk of an imbalance in the diet and can impact your metabolism further, making it difficult to lose weight and cut stubborn fat from the body.

Furthermore, there is a tendency to look for alternatives while shopping for allergen-free items; but, again, if you don't study the labels carefully, you could end up consuming more hidden sugar, extra calories, and unnecessary fats that could again lead to weight gain and many other health issues.

Reduced Physical Activities

Allergies can cause severe health conditions, like rashes, swelling, and itching. If not treated well, allergy symptoms can cause a huge setback in leading a regular life. It is natural to feel exhausted when you are constantly feeling dizzy, nauseated, sneezing, itching, down with the flu, and the like. When you are not in your best health, working out or even running your everyday errands can seem like a mammoth task. Imagine a situation where you have nasal congestion and itching at the same time. It would be almost impossible to even go for a walk!

Fatigue, difficulty breathing, and the anxiety caused by allergies can be reasons enough to make you feel burdened to take a step ahead and start exercising. To maintain and lose weight, along with a healthy diet, staying physically active is a must. However, if you are prone to food sensitivity and allergies, then the symptoms might make it more of a challenge to stick to a workout regimen and strive to get in better shape.

Emotional Eating

Consider falling sick because of some food allergy, and to top it all, refrain from eating something you find delicious and lip-smackingly good! Every time you crave something, instead of simply placing an order and eating, you have to go through the pain of checking with the restaurant about the ingredients and the labels on the food. It can be a tiring process and enough reason to feel frustrated and exhausted in the long run.

Just like binge-watching a TV series is a way to kill boredom, so is emotional eating a way to cope with the frustration of constant allergies that are a hindrance to leading a normal life. Staying at home and binging on food in an effort to feel better can be a great way to escape reality for some time. However, in that process, emotional eating increases your calorie intake and can be enough to make you gain weight in the long run.

Food allergies can impact many other aspects of your life, not just your health. For instance, socializing with friends and family may seem like a task because of not being able to participate and freely eat anything from the plate. Food is an essential part of gatherings and is also a medium through which people bond. Being unable to eat out freely can adversely affect your social relationships and even your self-esteem.

Habit replacement is a great thing to work toward if you are an emotional eater. When you crave food and eat that food, you are getting an internal shot of dopamine. This is the "high" you feel from emotional eating. If you replace the habit with a healthier habit that gives you the same high (shot of dopamine), then you end up with a comparable coping mechanism that has a healthier outcome. Try cleaning out a cabinet, painting your nails, calling a friend, doing jumping jacks, or anything that sounds fun to you and takes about the same amount of time as eating a snack, about three to five minutes. Make a list of these and go to your list the next time you want to eat due to emotion rather than hunger.

Medications

One of the most common medications given for allergic reactions is called antihistamine. Medicines like Allegra, Benadryl, Claritin, and Zyrtec are some of the antihistamines used all over the globe to counter allergic reactions. These medications are highly effective and powerful, but they also have a few adverse effects, like weight gain.

In some of the medicines prescribed by doctors, there is a substantial quantity of steroids, which can manage symptoms caused by allergic responses but can also make losing weight a bit difficult. Also, most antihistamine medicines are known to create a drowsy feeling and act as an effective sedative. The heaviness and sleepy feeling can make it very difficult for you to go out for physical activity, yet regular workouts are necessary to burn calories and achieve optimal health.

So, losing weight while dealing with allergies can be a difficult task. However, with a little more awareness, conscious eating, and regular exercise, you can deal with these issues and strive to achieve your best health and fitness. Choose from foods you have no allergy or sensitivity to in order to get closer to the flat belly you.

Chapter 5:

Prioritizing Bowel Regularity

Time to talk poop! Probably got a giggle out of you, but it's a little talked about topic, and we gotta hit it here when addressing flat belly goals. Bowel movements are absolutely important for your general health.

When this topic pops up, it's cringy for many of us, and we would rather push even the slightest conversations mentioning "poop" aside. First, no worries, because it is a very natural process and has to be equally paid attention to as we would for the rest of our bodily functions. So, bowel movements must be understood and carefully studied for greater awareness of how they affect how we live our lives for maximum vitality.

Understanding the Importance of Regular Bowel Movements

We don't waste a minute appreciating our lungs and respiratory system for the air we are able to breathe (especially if you have been sick and congested or struggled to breathe recently), and very rightly so because that keeps us living. However, if I start thanking my regular bowel movements for keeping me healthy, I bet everyone will be rather shocked and maybe disgusted as well. LOL! Our holistic health depends on various factors, and to feel healthy and fit, every organ and aspect of our systems should function at peak levels. But I am not exaggerating here: Regular bowel movements are vital for overall health and definitely for a flat stomach.

So, what is considered a regular healthy bowel movement? This can have various answers, as the frequency of bowel movements is not the same for everyone. For example, some may have bowel movements every day and, sometimes, even twice a day. For some, it might be an occurrence only three times or once a week. So, according to your unique bowel patterns, you can understand what falls within your general norms.

Here are some of the reasons why regular bowel movements are necessary:

- **Removing of waste:** Simply put, bowel movements help the system to empty the intestine and get rid of the waste and toxins present. It is a very integral process for human health. It flushes out the toxins and harmful substances from the colon.

- **Preventing diseases:** Irregular bowel movements can cause severe discomfort, the formation of gas, bloating, and constipation issues. These issues can further lay the groundwork for several other diseases, like colorectal issues, hemorrhoids, abdominal pain, a weakened immune system, and, in some cases, cancer. Difficulty passing stool regularly can also cause rectal bleeding, anal fissures, nausea, and excessive pain. However, regular bowel movements can help prevent such conditions.

From toxin removal to improving the quality of life, regular and healthy-sized or shaped bowel movements can be extremely beneficial for your wellness.

Role in Digestive Health and Flat Belly Goals

Your bowel movement patterns say a lot about your digestive and gut health. Regular and smooth passing indicates that the food consumed is well broken down in the system, the nutrients are well absorbed in the body, and the gut feels healthy due to the presence of good microbes, making your immunity strong. In addition, this can be advantageous for those trying to maintain their weight and, in many cases, lose some weight as well.

An interesting study shows how your bowel can give a clear insight into why you are not able to lose belly fat! A study was done on the bacterial diversity of 3,600 bowel samples from 1,300 twins. Their visceral body fat and subcutaneous fat were measured, and the result found through comparison was that the more diverse and variant their microbiome was, the lower their risk of getting obese and having visceral fat (Mackenzie, 2016). Through this research, we see that your gut health is directly responsible for helping maintain weight. While one study may not be definitive, there is definitely no harm in giving it some importance and taking good care by eating right.

One question that instantly pops up in this case is: Does your bowel movement really affect your weight-loss effort? The answer can be a bit complex. There are many people who experience a drop in their weight after a bout of vomiting and diarrhea. To be precise, if you check your weight after a day or two of having diarrhea, the drop in weight that you see on the scale is all about the water weight and not at all about any permanent fat loss. The two types of fat we have in our bodies are visceral and subcutaneous fat. The former is the fat that is gathered around your organs, and thus in the waist, and can be very dangerous for overall health, and the latter is mostly the fat that is beneath the skin (Walters, 2018).

As we have already discussed in the previous chapters, sticking to macro counting and maintaining a healthy lifestyle with regular exercise are the most effective ways to reduce fat and lose weight. A healthy colon with no gas or waste stuck can make the belly appear and feel flat. However, with constipation and digestive issues, you can feel bloated, which is why regular bowel movement is so important. Having said that, it is true that regular bowel movements can help you stay comfortable and even feel light, but losing weight by pooping a lot quickly really does not make any sense for a long-term weight-loss and weight-maintenance strategy.

Signs of Healthy Bowel Function

Two of the indicators for understanding healthy bowel function are its consistency and color.

Stool Color

The color, texture, and consistency of your stool can depend on various simple factors, like the type of food you ate the day before or the amount of fluids you drank. There could be many underlying causes for a certain abnormality if it stays the same for a prolonged period. However, the color of your stool can say a lot about your health.

- **Brown:** All brown-colored stools are considered normal. The bile formed in the liver mixes with the digested food in the intestine, which results in a brown color.

- **Yellow:** A yellow-colored stool with a slight odor and grease could indicate some bacterial infections and digestive issues. It is mainly seen in babies who breastfeed.

- **Green:** Green stool could be caused by medications, like iron supplements and antibiotics. Consumption of green vegetables and drinks could also be the reason for the color. It could be caused by particular foods or drinks that passed through the gut and did not digest well, indicating a gastrointestinal disorder as well.

- **Red:** It is usually the food and drinks you consume that can cause red stool. However, if the stool is consistently red, then that could be because of some bleeding in the gastrointestinal tract.

- **Black:** A few medicines, like iron supplements, can cause the stool to turn black. Similarly, certain foods, like blueberries, blood sausages, black licorice, etc., can cause the same. However, if there is no such food consumed, it could hint at an underlying condition, like bleeding in the intestines.

If you notice that you are consistently getting such colored stool without consuming any food or drinks that could possibly cause it, you should visit your doctor for a thorough checkup (Alzayer, 2022).

Stool Consistency

Regular bowel movements indicate good gastrointestinal health. Irregular bowel movements, at times, do not pose any immediate harm; but if continued for a prolonged amount of time, it can be problematic.

According to the Bristol stool chart, there are seven different types of stool consistency, and each could indicate a certain condition. Let us look at them in detail:

- **Type 1:** This type of stool is hard, separate, and, in the form of lumps, feels like constipation and can be quite difficult to pass.

- **Type 2:** This type of stool looks like sausage but is a bit lumpy. It could indicate that you are constipated.

- **Type 3:** This type of stool also looks like sausage, but it has cracks on the surface area.

- **Type 4:** This type of stool also looks like sausage but is very soft and smooth.

- **Type 5:** This type of stool has clear-cut edges and is in the form of soft blobs, which are very easy to pass.

- **Type 6:** This type of stool is mushy, fluffy in texture, and very easy to pass.

- **Type 7:** This type of stool is entirely in liquid form.

Dr. Ken Heaton, assisted by 66 volunteers from the University of Bristol, generated this chart in 1997 (WebMD Editorial Contributors, 2015). There has been remarkable documented information that has helped in understanding the complexities of health with regard to the bowel style and movements of a person.

Factors Influencing Bowel Regularity

Bowel movements and their regularity vary from person to person. If you have watched *The Big Bang Theory*, you know that it is a fantastic sitcom where the lead character

Sheldon is a scientist and is extremely particular about his bathroom schedule. He is a genius who insists on keeping this bathroom schedule because it is true: Your habits and routines play a major role in deciding at what time and how frequently you will poop. Although a little nutty, he wasn't wrong!

Many factors contribute to frequent or fewer bowel movements. Here are a few primary factors influencing bowel regularity:

Dietary Fiber and Hydration

Studies show that around 27% of adults suffer from symptoms of constipation, bloating, gas, and digestion-related conditions caused mainly by increasing age and a more sedentary lifestyle (Petre, 2017).

The foods you consume play a key role in how your bowel movement will be. Dietary fiber is an integral part of a well-rounded diet. It is great for accelerating bowel movements and also helps prevent constipation problems. Dietary fibers are divided into two categories:

- **Insoluble fiber:** This type of fiber accelerates the frequency and bulk of stool.

- **Soluble fiber:** This type of fiber helps regulate blood sugar and cholesterol levels.

Eating fiber-rich food can significantly help in regulating bowel movements. Drinking enough water and keeping your body hydrated at all times is also vital. Water helps digest food, makes the stool softer, and prevents the risk of constipation.

Lifestyle Habits and Stress Management

Your dietary lifestyle habits have an impact on your social life, job, health, and happiness in general. The condition of your digestive system is impacted by the food you eat, your physical exertion level, and your degree of stress, which might result in bowel habits that are inconsistent.

If you are facing issues with digestive health and bowel movement issues, you should make an effort to stay away from the following:

- **Red meat:** Red meat contains proteins and several micronutrients, but it is extremely low in fiber. This is one of the reasons why the consumption of red meat in excess can increase the risk of severe constipation. It is heavy for your system, can cause bulkiness in the stool, and can cause irregular bowel movements. By making a conscious effort, you can opt for plant-based protein sources, like lentils, legumes, beans, etc., instead of devouring a heavy steak if it is causing bowel issues for you.

- **Alcohol:** Drinking an excessive amount of alcohol can lead to dehydration, which can further cause severe health conditions. With dehydration, the risk of constipation increases as the frequency of urination also slows down. However, the effects of alcohol can have different consequences for different people. For example, in many cases, after drinking for the whole night or in large quantities, some may even get stomach upset and diarrhea.

- **Dairy products:** Studies were done by replacing cow's milk with soy milk and giving it to children suffering from chronic constipation. It was seen that cow's milk aggravated their constipation, and when the milk was changed to soy milk, their condition improved, and they got relief. The protein found in cow's milk can cause mild to severe complications if you have digestive and food intolerance issues (Crowley et al., 2008).

- **Processed grains:** Flour used in pasta, white bread, and noodles is mostly processed and contains very little fiber, which can cause constipation and other digestive issues. This is one of the reasons why nutritionists often suggest whole grains as an alternative to processed grains, where the bran and fiber present in the grains are removed during processing. Fiber helps in bowel movement, but again, it depends on the health and condition of the patient.

- **Gluten:** There are many who are intolerant to gluten, which is a protein found in grains like barley, wheat, rye, triticale, and kamut. Especially for a person suffering from celiac disease, consumption of gluten-laden food can cause more intolerance issues and inflame their immune system. Chronic constipation is another adverse effect that could result from consumption of gluten.

- **Stress:** Studies show how stress can adversely affect a person's overall health, including digestive and bowel movement dysfunction. When a person faces stress, their body releases a hormone called epinephrine as a response. This diverts the blood flow to other organs from the intestine, and the intestinal movement slows down, causing constipation. The permeability of the intestine also increases, causing a feeling of fullness and discomfort in the abdomen (Petre, 2020).

In some cases, people do not even realize that the food and drinks they are consuming cause bowel-related problems. With the increase in access to takeout and fast food joints, we, as a society, are consuming more processed food without even realizing it. For example, in the case of mass-baked brown bread, some buy it thinking there is no flour in it. This could be a serious concern for those struggling with gluten allergies, because if you check the label, you will notice that there is white flour in it, which, in my opinion, makes brown bread lose its purpose. Your lifestyle plays a huge role in how you feel physically and mentally. More so, if you have food intolerance and allergy issues, you must all the more be aware of what you consume. Reading the labels on food items and being aware of what makes your bowel regular can also help you feel better in the long run, in addition to helping keep your stomach from protruding.

Practical Strategies for Improving Bowel Regularity

Diet Modifications and Hydration Practices

Sometimes, health issues are such that regardless of how much you try, you may not be able to avoid them altogether. The best you can do is find ways to keep them at bay as much as possible. Imagine reaching an age where it becomes extremely difficult to reverse many ailments and diseases. To prevent that from happening, efforts must be made *now* to make dietary modifications and increase hydration, along with adopting a healthy lifestyle.

Here are a few tips that can help you do it in an easy way:

Increase Fiber-Rich Foods in Your Diet

Americans are said to consume quite less than the recommended daily dose of fiber, which for women is 25 grams and for men is 38 grams per day. Beans, broccoli, berries, avocados, whole grains, popcorn, lentils, chia seeds, dried fruits, apples, nuts, potatoes, split peas, chickpeas, quinoa, almonds, pears, oats, bananas, carrots, beets, artichoke, Brussels sprouts, kale, spinach, tomatoes, sweet potatoes, dark chocolates, etc., are some of the sources of fiber. However, it has to be noted that increasing fiber in your diet quickly is not recommended. You should gradually introduce or increase the portion of fiber-rich foods in your diet. The correct amount of fiber intake can help with weight loss, diabetes, and improving bowel movements (Gunnars, 2020).

Include Probiotics in Your Diet

As we know, gut health and its microbiome have a major role to play in keeping the gastrointestinal tract and digestive health healthy and functioning. The good bacteria in your system not only help improve immunity but also improve digestive functions, making bowel movements smooth, too. A healthy gut also helps you maintain and lose weight by increasing your metabolism as a whole. Lifelong Metabolic Center has a fantastic probiotic available over the counter. Look for a USP label to ensure probiotics have been quality tested by a third party that had nothing to gain from the outcome of the testing.

Check for Food Sensitivity

Food sensitivity is one of the many reasons for getting bowel issues like constipation. For example, when milk protein is not digested well in the system, it causes flatulence, diarrhea, or even constipation. Eliminate or replace any food item that causes you discomfort and digestion issues. Using excessive oil while cooking or having too many dairy products can affect your health in the long run or give *you* the runs in the short run.

Avoid Processed Food

Most processed foods contain high levels of sodium, flour, preservatives, and artificial colors and are generally very low in fiber. Consuming processed food in excess can cause many health issues, like constipation, high cholesterol, and blood pressure issues. Regular intake of such food can heavily affect your metabolism and cause weight gain.

Eat Prunes

Prunes are rich in polyphenols, fructans, fiber, probiotics, and sorbitol. They are exceptionally good for bowel movements. They have laxative properties and are said to relieve constipation and also help regulate stool volume and frequency of bowel movements. But again, don't overdo these, or you can end up with gas and/or diarrhea.

A Few Herbs and Tips That Help

There are numerous natural treatments and supplements available to help reduce conditions of bowel movements, like diarrhea, constipation, and many other digestive issues.

For diarrhea

- Bovine colostrum is the milk produced immediately and for a few days after a cow gives birth. It is rich in antibodies, cytokines, and growth factors, which help treat diarrhea in adults.

- Berberine is a medicinal plant with microbial properties that helps fight viruses, fungi, and bacteria and also helps with diarrhea.

- Similarly, chamomile and berry leaf teas are beneficial in reducing inflammation in the gut. Ginger can help with diarrhea caused by IBS.

For constipation

- Senna tea is a traditional herb used to clean the colon.

- Cascara sagrada falls under unregulated herbal supplements but has been used over the years for relieving constipation.

- Amalaka powder is used in Ayurvedic medicine, is beneficial for digestion, and is said to ease constipation as well.

- Triphala is also an herb used in Ayurvedic medicine and is said to have a laxative effect. It can help reduce bloating, abdominal pain, and bowel issues.

- Peppermint oil can be great for digestive health. It relaxes the gut muscles and reduces abdominal pain.

- Artichoke leaf extract is very effective in regulating bowel issues, especially constipation problems.

- Aloe vera is a plant that helps to reduce the effects of IBS, diabetes, constipation, and many skin issues as well.

- Slippery elm is an herbal medicine that has been used by Native Americans to treat many health issues. It has a calming effect on the intestines and eases diarrhea or constipation.

For dehydration

Bowel issues like constipation can be caused by dehydration. Many times, when the food you consume lacks water content, the large intestine will make an effort to pull water from the waste instead. This can cause hard stool and constipation issues, further causing pain during bowel movements

Drinking more water and eating foods with a high water content can help prevent dehydration. Your body loses a lot of water during and after strenuous physical activities, like exercise and even walking daily, especially on hot days. Through sweat and urine, the body loses water, and if not replenished with more water intake, there can be serious dehydration issues.

Drink half of your body weight in ounces per day. Drink enough water and avoid caffeinated drinks. If the dehydration is a bit more than normal, then having fluids with electrolytes can be very helpful as well. Gatorade has recently come out with some lighter versions with less sugar and all-natural ingredients. You can even boil a banana with the ends cut off and drink the "tea" to get your electrolytes back in check as well.

Incorporating Physical Activity and Stress-Reduction Techniques

Stress is a part of modern-day existence. There are so many factors that you deal with every single day of your life that can impact your mind and health in many different ways. When your body and mind are not in sync, stress can take over your holistic wellness.

Physical activities play a significant role in managing stress. This happens because when your body is physically active and moving, blood circulation increases, which positively affects your brain health. Endorphins, also referred to as "feel-good hormones," help reduce stress and give a positive "high" after physical activity, which is one of the primary reasons why most people feel happy after a good workout.

By incorporating regular exercises and a few stress-reduction methods, you can regulate many health conditions—including bowel irregularities.

Here are a few benefits exercises can bring:

- Studies show that regular exercise can enhance your immunity, reduce inflammation, and decrease the risk of getting several diseases. With exercise, blood and lymph flow increase and so does your immune cell circulation.

- Regular exercise helps reduce the risk of cardiovascular diseases and even bone health conditions.

- Physical activities can cause a slight alteration in antibodies and white blood cells, which are the immune system cells of the body that help fight against diseases.

- With regular workouts and physical activities, bacteria are flushed out of the system through the airways, which helps prevent flu-type symptoms/conditions.

- After physical activity, body temperature slightly increases, which is said to prevent the spread of bacteria and infections, similar to how fever fights against infections.

- Stress can cause severe illnesses, but with regular exercise, the production of cortisol, a stress hormone, decreases, resulting in a lowered risk of ailments caused by stress. There are direct correlations between a reduction in cortisol and a reduction in belly fat, too.

- Exercise can make you feel better and happier! Physical activities help produce endorphins, the hormones responsible for reducing pain and inducing happiness. This is one of the reasons why after a good workout, you feel uplifted and positive.

- A study showed how regular exercise for about six weeks can reduce tiredness for people who reportedly complained about fatigue for a very long time (Loy et al., 2013). This shows how regular exercise can help increase your energy levels.

- Regular exercise is said to reduce hypertension and can also reduce the risk of developing cardiovascular conditions.

- Exercise is effective in reducing constipation and regulating bowel movements. With exercises like aerobics and cardio, your heart and breathing rate increase because the contraction of muscles in the intestine is increased making it easier to help excrete stools easily (Fulghum, 2007).

- Exercising and keeping yourself physically active throughout the day can help you sleep better at night.

I understand that working out at a gym or going out for a run may not be always feasible. However, the key is moving your body as much as you can! Regardless of how busy your schedule is or where you are, ensure that you give yourself a minimum of 20 to 30 minutes each day to do some stretches, on-the-spot jogging, yoga poses, or any convenient exercise. Inactivity is a major culprit for weight gain, and if it is combined with excessive stress and exhaustion, it becomes especially problematic for your belly fat as well.

The American Heart Association recommends a minimum of 150 minutes of moderate exercise a week. Being physically active can divert your attention from stressful thoughts and situations and make you feel better and more positive. The more physically active you are, the more connected you will feel to the rhythm of your body and movements. Exercising can not only make you physically fit but can also keep your mind calm and relaxed.

Exercises like biking, hiking, brisk walking, jogging, swimming, climbing stairs, water aerobics, dancing, rowing, playing a sport, and other forms of aerobic exercise are extremely beneficial in managing stress, improving health, and reducing weight. If you ever feel anxious or if anger is bubbling up inside of you, try taking a quiet walk outside. In no time, you will sense how your stress fades, and you will feel energetic and much happier (Madel, 2012).

Tips to Reduce Stress in General

When we are young, we don't have to think much about taking care of ourselves. Our bodies are strong and energetic. With growing age and added responsibilities in life, our physical and mental health tend to take a back seat to the hustle and bustle of middle-aged lifestyles. Slowly, stress and exhaustion creep in and often leave behind several health complications before we realize it. We don't feel old mentally, but we start to *feel* old physically long before we should. If we start to pay attention *now* and take action *now*, we can stretch our vitality much, much longer.

This is one of the reasons why anyone, regardless of age, can and should start a self-care routine and attempt every approach to reduce stress in any form. We all know by now how excessive stress can cause health issues and can lead to many bowel issues as well.

Here are a few tips that can guide you to help reduce stress:

- **Exercise regularly:** Regular activities can keep your mind stress free and happy. The hormones produced after your body goes through a workout can make you feel happy and relieve stress and anxiety.

- **Follow a diet plan:** A well-rounded diet free from processed and artificial foods can add more benefits to your health and keep your body and mind clean and healthy. Stress and anxiety can cause many hindrances to your diet routine. For example, cases like binge eating or eating less due to stress can cause severe nutrient deficiency and, in many cases, bloating and weight gain or loss issues. Following a healthy diet plan is essential for staying low stress.

- **Reduce screen time:** Excessive use of gadgets can cause anxiety, frustration, and low psychological well-being. By reducing screen time, you can get more time for yourself and sleep better at night, too.

- **Remember self-care:** Prioritizing your health and well-being is the best way to detox and de-stress your mind and body. Make time for yourself and try activities you enjoy. For example, read a book, light scented candles, take a relaxing bath, get a massage, take a walk, practice yoga, or do something that works for you and makes you feel refreshed, renewed, and restored.

- **Journal:** It is normal to feel the desire to let your emotions and anxieties out when you are overwhelmed and overloaded. It might not always be feasible or even the best course of action. So, keeping a journal can be a great outlet. Before going to bed, you might write about how your mental and physical health has changed over the day. By doing this, you will feel less stressed and will be able to subsequently identify all of your behavioral patterns and discover appropriate potential solutions.

- **Limit caffeine and alcohol:** The caffeine present in coffee, chocolate, tea, and energy drinks is known to stimulate your brain. Excessive consumption of caffeine can cause anxiety and can also cause insomnia. Cutting back on such caffeinated drinks and switching to drinking more water and herbal teas can be a better option to help reduce stress. Similarly, reducing the intake of alcohol can also help in reducing stress and anxiety.

- **Surround yourself with loved ones:** One study showed how young adults tend to suffer from depression, loneliness, and stress symptoms when they receive very little or no support from their friends, family, and partners (Lee et al., 2020). Spending time and doing things that you love with those you love (and like being around) can uplift your mood and fill your spirit with positivity and happiness. This can be an effective way to curb stress and anxiety.

- **Avoid procrastination:** Without a doubt, overthinking is a cause of stress, but more than that, a habit of procrastination can be a problematic issue that can cause stress, too. For example, when you decide to do something later, the thought of doing it and completing it will keep circling your mind, and eventually, the more you extend, the longer you will feel stressed about it. Avoiding procrastination decreases the amount of time that task is draining your mental energy.

- **Learn to say "no":** The burden of doing something when you don't want to or feel up for it can be negative for your mind. The stress you get from saying "yes" to someone or something when you don't mean it or want it can make you restless and frustrated. Saying a clear "no" to things you do not want can clear your headspace and also help you feel better and less responsible for anything not needed in your life.

- **Try yoga:** A great way to counter stress is by practicing yoga, the age-old form of exercise known for its benefits for your holistic health. There are different poses and asanas in yoga for every body part and a variety of health conditions. I even started doing face yoga recently. It is an amazing way to drain lymph in your face, neck, and shoulders; increase circulation; and perhaps even avoid a wrinkle or two. The jury is still out on that one. Check back with me in a few years, and we will see. From relieving body aches and losing weight to healing the body and calming the mind, yoga can boost your health and well-being.

- **Meditate:** Mindful meditation has been practiced by people for thousands of years. The benefits of meditation, especially mindful meditation, can help your mind in many ways. It can balance your mind and body and sync them so beautifully that your body becomes less stressed and healthier over time.

- **Go outside:** Nature is the ultimate healer! Studies show how spending even as little as 10 minutes in nature can help your physical and mental well-being (Meredith et al., 2020). Taking some time out and spending it in the outdoors can not only help you feel better, but it can also give you a whole new perspective. It helps to enjoy the environment around you and appreciate the beauty of nature.

- **Engage in touch:** Having positive contact with someone, particularly physically, like a long hug or cuddle, can help soothe your mind and reduce stress. Human touch is said to be very healing and has a relieving effect of calming your mind and body. This is primarily caused by the production of oxytocin, which helps lower the stress hormone cortisol, which, in turn, has many health benefits.

- **Breathe:** Stress can cause severe changes in your mental and physical condition. The human body responds to stress and gets into a fight-or-flight mode to cope with it. An increase in stress and cortisol levels can lead to health conditions like heart palpitations, constricted blood vessels, and fast breathing. The way we breathe has a lot to do with how our bodies function. Through awareness and careful practice of different types of breathing exercises, you can feel more relaxed and rejuvenated. Some effective breathing exercises are diaphragmatic, alternate nostril, paced, and box breathing. When you are aware of your breath, you will feel more alive and conscious of the present, which will help divert your mind from stressful thoughts. Take slow and deep breaths and feel the air enter your system through your nose. Gradually fill your lungs, and when your lungs and belly fully expand, release the air slowly through your mouth. This can be one of the easiest and fastest ways to feel calm and relaxed.

- **Ask for help:** Asking for help is the bravest thing you can do! Too often, people keep their tension and worries to themselves and then face unnecessary struggles. The stress caused by mental health issues can be huge, so it is very important to acknowledge the existence of any mental health issues you are facing. Sometimes, we need help dealing with our own struggles, and sometimes we need to know how to best help those around us cope without absorbing it ourselves. Instead of being embarrassed, take the help of the people you are close to and also seek professional help if and when needed. Therapy and counseling sessions can help you understand what you are dealing with and, in turn, help you find what you need.

Conclusion

As we near the end of our journey together, it seems plausible to say that with knowledge, purpose, and the will to make a few healthy changes, you are capable of accomplishing unimaginably great things! Through this book, I embarked on a mission to reach out to those who have had doubts about their fitness and overall well-being and are searching for some great tips and tricks to achieve a flat(er) belly. The way our bodies act and react is something we hardly sit and think about in this era of hustle and bustle. I'm sure you would agree with me when I say that our health has taken a big hit from living this way—too fast and too furious.

A sedentary lifestyle, which is commonplace for many, has increased the risk of several health concerns, including problems with unhealthy weight and weight gain. Though everyone *can* work to achieve and maintain the size they want, it isn't always easy. It is also true that the larger your waistline, the higher the chances of disease. Everything we do is associated in some way or another with how we feel. It is not about reaching for stereotypical beauty standards by encouraging you to shed a few inches from your waist; it is about awareness of health and fitness that makes me say that it is better to work and sweat now and lose those inches than face problems due to lack of vitality later in life.

Summing Up the Journey

From the start of this book, the guiding aspects have focused on five factors for fighting belly flab. If we look back at the journey we have made together since way back on page 1, you will notice that the concept of weight loss is not simply about decreasing the numbers on the scale; it is about how healthy your mind and body are and the quality of life through your later years as well.

We started off discussing the salt we consume and how to avoid it or get the right amount for you, and then we gradually moved to topics like embracing healthy fats in your diet, managing gaseous food, avoiding food sensitivities, and achieving regular bowel movements. Losing belly fat was not the only focus; we discussed more about all the underlying factors you may need to address first.

In addition to demonstrating how to get a flat belly, I have tried to paint a clearer picture of the whys and hows behind each tip. Spot reduction of weight or fat is quite difficult, if not impossible, so when focusing on reducing belly fat, you must also make an effort to adopt a healthy lifestyle with a dedication to consistent dietary changes and regular movement.

Key Takeaways

Here are our Five Fast Flat Belly Facts in a nutshell:

Sodium Sensitivity

We have learned about the various aspects of sodium sensitivity and its impact on our lives. Now, you'll be better able to address your water retention difficulties. Next time you weigh yourself and see the scale jump up, do not fret! Double-check if it could be due to sodium; don't assume you need a whole new diet plan. A root-cause analysis of any issue is critical since it can avert a plethora of unnecessary concerns and worries.

Sodium sensitivity can jeopardize your overall wellness, possibly causing hypertension, cardiovascular conditions, and even stroke. Your effort to shed inches from your waist may be going well, but without realizing it, the added salt you sprinkle on your foods every time you eat could be stopping you from getting in the shape you want as quickly as you want.

Constant feelings of being bloated and puffy are not pleasant, and once you understand that it might be sodium causing these symptoms, you can take measures and make necessary lifestyle and diet changes. Often, it's enough to monitor your salt intake to address water retention issues and other ailments. However, overdoing anything may be harmful, so instead of eliminating salt completely, limit your intake to a minimum. With conscious decisions like this, you will soon see a difference in your health and weight.

Embracing Healthy Fats

While there is a widespread fear of "fat" in the world around us, don't forget that "good fats" can do wonders for your overall health! Fats are essential for your body to function at an optimal level. It helps regulate cholesterol levels, reduces inflammation, optimizes cognitive abilities, improves liver health, strengthens bones, improves skin condition, reduces sleep issues, regulates blood sugar levels, and even helps maintain weight.

If your main goal is to lose extra weight, then—contrary to what some people believe—consuming healthy fats can be advantageous. Science shows that a decent amount of healthy monosaturated fats in your daily diet can make weight loss much easier. A high-fat diet to reduce weight can work great for those who need more fats in their balanced diet, too. The Lifelong Metabolic Center Program offers a custom macro count with a simple cheek swab to tell you the exact right amount of fats for your specific body. Contact us if you are interested in losing weight or just seeing the right amounts of food and exercise for *you*.

A lack of knowledge can create countless misconceptions. Don't deprive yourself of good fats thinking that all fats are the same! You need the right information to take care of your health and wellness properly.

For example, I remember the days when I would feel bloated and, in fact, even gain substantial fat around my waist and thighs. My first reaction would be to panic, and

I would cater to all the wrong but quick fixes to solve this problem. Little did I realize that tossing out the nutritious almond butter jar in an attempt to lose weight would be one of the worst choices I made! If I had gotten the appropriate advice from an expert when I was growing up or in my teens, I would have known how to boost my body acceptance and keep active without giving up the foods I actually loved eating. The bottom line is that you don't have to give up on fats to shed fat from your body! Regardless of your age, being consistent with good, sensible choices will keep you strong and help you achieve the life you have envisioned for yourself long term.

The Buzz on Bloat

Coming back to the smelly topic of gas and gaseous food, one thing that stands out is recognizing the most common food items that tend to fill you up with gas and cause several painful side effects along with it. Gas and acidity issues can create a lot of hurdles in your everyday life. Consider the following scenario: You have a long flight with friends, and you start feeling gassy and bloated from the night before. And, to top it all off, you are freaking out you won't be *able* to hold it all in (like the poor dude on the news lately who had diarrhea and the flight had to land)! These scenarios can be avoided if you know which foods cause you distress from your food journaling.

There could be days when an antacid pill or Beano could do the trick and make you feel better in a jiffy. There could also be days when it takes exceptionally long for the gas to pass through your system, causing excessive discomfort and pain. Managing gaseous food can be tricky but is definitely not rocket science. With the help of this book, you can learn more about the digestive processes and also easily identify the various food items that could cause flatulence and chronic gas. I've mentioned in detail the different medical issues associated with gastrointestinal disorders and the various ways to prevent gas formation. With a careful selection of food and drinks, you can manage gas issues in very simple ways. Avoiding gaseous foods is an easy way to get a flatter stomach.

Food Sensitivities and Such

While it might be obvious to avoid a food you are allergic to because it gives you a rash, swelling, or difficulty breathing, sometimes figuring out food sensitivities can be much more elusive. A great way to test for these is a reverse elimination diet. By avoiding foods you are sensitive to, you can stop unnecessary belly bloat.

Poop Power

Finally, as gross as it may sound, we fixated quite a bit on bowel movements. The sensitivity around the entire "poop" discussion is real, and people prefer to not mention it, let alone discuss it out in the open. Here, I have made an effort to understand bowel movements in the most normal way, like the way we would discuss our respiratory or nervous systems. One of my goals is to create maximum awareness among my patients and followers—regardless of age, gender, or body size—to come forward and learn about their bodies.

The nature of bowel movements plays a major role in our physical and also our mental health. The food we eat and the way it gets processed and digested in the system are imperative for providing nutrients and energy throughout the body. Irregularity and difficulty in bowel movements can adversely affect your general well-being, including your mood!

Parting Wisdom

Our journey to health and happiness includes fresh knowledge, old experiences, wisdom, obstacles, and a myriad of treasures because of our years of life. When we look in the mirror, we may just see a double chin, some gray hair strands, or perhaps a button on the midriff of our shirts that has loosened due to an increasing belly. Try to also see the beautiful, amazing machine that is your body. Appreciate your abilities and gifts, too.

Whether your goal is to lose weight and flatten your stomach, to look the best you've ever looked, or to feel the healthiest you've ever felt, one thing to remember is that having the correct understanding of our physical and mental health definitely helps. Especially in this age of widely available, yet not always correct, information. From learning the effects of consuming sodium and increasing your intake of healthy fats to understanding your relationship with various food items, the way a simple nut can make you look like a puffer fish, adopting a healthy lifestyle, and understanding the true nature of your poop, we have covered it all, and I hope this knowledge will help you navigate your health issues and maybe gave you an extra smile or two here or there along the way.

Through this book, I hope you will realize the importance of being your healthiest self. Additionally, every time you think about working toward a flatter belly, may it be to feel and become as healthy as you can be. The point is not to get a large amount of "likes" and validation from social media or acceptance from your critics. Rather, it is all about loving yourself, being grateful for the health and vitality you have, and simply making the best effort to stay healthy for the longest period of time. The work you put in now can give you more years in your life and life in your years!

Thank you for taking this journey towards a healthier you with me. I hope this book has provided you with valuable insights, practical tips, and the motivation you need to achieve your weight loss goals.

As an author, there's nothing more rewarding than hearing how my work has made a difference in your life. Your feedback not only helps me grow as a writer but also assists future readers in discovering this book and finding their own path to success.

If you've found this book helpful, I would be incredibly grateful if you could take a moment to share your thoughts by leaving a review on Amazon. Your honest review can inspire others to take the first step towards their own transformation and can help make this book more visible to those who need it most.

Here's how you can leave a review:

1. **Go to the Book's Amazon Page**: https://www.amazon.com/review/review-your-purchases/?asin=B0D3ZK83X4
2. **Share Your Experience**: Your review doesn't need to be long—just a few sentences about how the book helped you or what you enjoyed most.
3. **Rate the Book**: If you found the book useful, a five-star rating is appreciated, but feel free to be honest about your experience.

Every review counts and makes a big difference! Whether you share what you loved, what could be improved, or simply a quick note of encouragement, your feedback is invaluable.

Thank you once again for your support. Together, we're building a community of individuals committed to better health and well-being. I look forward to hearing from you and wish you continued success on your weight loss journey!

Love,

Dr. Amanda Borre, D.C.

References

Alzayer, G. (2022, May 27). *What healthy bowel movements look like, and when to call the doctor.* Medstar Health. https://www.medstarhealth.org/blog/healthy-bowel-movements-look-like

Ball, J. (2022, August 13). *7 ways to add 10 grams of healthy fat to your meals.* Eating Well. https://www.eatingwell.com/article/7993588/ways-to-add-healthy-fat-to-your-meals/

Berry, J. (2020, January 20). *18 ways to reduce bloating: Quick tips and long-term relief.* Medical News Today. https://www.medicalnewstoday.com/articles/322525

Brehm, B. J., Lattin, B. L., Summer, S. S., Boback, J. A., Gilchrist, G. M., Jandacek, R. J., & D'Alessio, D. A. (2008). *One-year comparison of a high-monounsaturated fat diet with a high-carbohydrate diet in type 2 diabetes.* Diabetes Care, *32*(2), 215–220. https://doi.org/10.2337/dc08-0687

Cianferoni, A. (2016). *Wheat allergy: diagnosis and management.* Journal of Asthma and Allergy, 13. https://doi.org/10.2147/jaa.s81550

Cording, J. (2018, December 9). *Want to avoid gas & bloating at holiday parties? Don't eat this food.* MBG

Food. https://www.mindbodygreen.com/articles/how-cruciferous-vegetables-can-cause-gas-and-bloating

Crowley, E., Williams, L., Roberts, T., Jones, P., & Dunstan, R. (2008). Evidence for a role of cow's milk consumption in chronic functional constipation in children: Systematic review of the literature from 1980 to 2006. *Nutrition & Dietetics*, *65*(1), 29–35. https://doi.org/10.1111/j.1747-0080.2007.00225.x

Dallas, M. E. (2023, April 7). *Home remedies to relieve gas and reduce bloating*. EverydayHealth. https://www.everydayhealth.com/excessive-gas/home-remedies-for-gas

Dicks, L. (2022). Gut bacteria and neurotransmitters. *Microorganisms*, *10*(9), 1838. https://doi.org/10.3390/microorganisms10091838

DiLonardo, M. (2018). *Gastroenteritis (stomach "flu")*. WebMD. https://www.webmd.com/digestive-disorders/gastroenteritis

Do allergies affect your gastro health? (2023, May 11). GI Associates & Endoscopy Center. https://gi.md/resources/articles/do-allergies-affect-your-gastro-health#

Dolan, E. W. (2023, June 4). *New research indicates visceral fat has a profoundly negative effect on cognitive abilities*. PsyPost.

https://www.psypost.org/2023/06/new-research-indicates-visceral-fat-has-a-profoundly-negative-effect-on-cognitive-abilities-164382

Eske, J. (2023, January 6). *Leaky gut syndrome: What it is, symptoms, and treatments.* https://www.medicalnewstoday.com/articles/326117#summary

Food allergy versus food intolerance. (2019, March 15). Allergy Insider. https://www.thermofisher.com/allergy/wo/en/living-with-allergies/food-allergies/food-allergy-vs-food-intolerance.html

Food allergy (2021, December 31). Mayo Clinic. https://www.mayoclinic.org/diseases-conditions/food-allergy/symptoms-causes/syc-20355095

Fluid retention (oedema). (2012). Better Health Channel. https://www.betterhealth.vic.gov.au/health/conditionsandtreatments/Fluid-retention-oedema

Fulghum, D. (2007a, June 22). *How drinking fluids can help you manage constipation.* WebMD; WebMD. https://www.webmd.com/digestive-disorders/water-a-fluid-way-to-manage-constipation

Fulghum, D. (2007b, June 25). *Exercise to ease constipation.* WebMD. https://www.webmd.com/digestive-disorders/exercise-curing-constipation-via-movement

Gastroesophageal reflux disease (GERD) (2023, January 4). Mayo Clinic. https://www.mayoclinic.org/diseases-conditions/gerd/symptoms-causes/syc-20361940

Godman, H. (2021, August 1). *Chronic gut inflammation: Coping with inflammatory bowel disease.* Harvard Health. https://www.health.harvard.edu/diseases-and-conditions/chronic-gut-inflammation-coping-with-inflammatory-bowel-disease

Gunnars, K. (2020, October 22). *22 high-fiber foods you should eat.* Healthline. https://www.healthline.com/nutrition/22-high-fiber-foods#faq

Gustafson, C. (2017). Bruce Lipton, Ph.D.: The jump from cell culture to consciousness. *Integrative Medicine (Encinitas, Calif.), 16*(6), 44–50. https://www.ncbi.nlm.nih.gov/pmc/articles/PMC6438088/

Haththotuwa, R. N., Wijeyaratne, C. N., & Senarath, U. (2020, January 1). *Chapter 1 - Worldwide epidemic of obesity* (T. A. Mahmood, S. Arulkumaran, & F. A. Chervenak, Eds.). ScienceDirect. https://www.sciencedirect.com/science/article/abs/pii/B9780128179215000011

Hill, M. (2018, November 16). *4 ways to improve your digestion if you're stressed.* Healthline.

https://www.healthline.com/health/four-ways-to-improve-your-gut-if-youre-stressed

How high blood pressure can affect your body. (2022, January 14). Mayo Clinic. https://www.mayoclinic.org/diseases-conditions/high-blood-pressure/in-depth/high-blood-pressure/art-20045868

How salt can impact your blood pressure, heart, and kidneys. (2017, June 15). Cleveland Clinic. https://health.clevelandclinic.org/kidneys-salt-and-blood-pressure-you-need-a-delicate-balance/

How to properly combine foods to improve digestive health. (2018, October 25). LiveFit. https://livefitfood.ca/blogs/news/how-to-properly-combine-foods-in-order-to-improve-digestive-health

Incredible benefits of Himalayan salt. (2023, October 2) Healthy Human. https://healthyhumanlife.com/blogs/news/benefits-of-himalayan-salt

Irritable bowel syndrome. (n.d.). Mayo Clinic. https://www.mayoclinic.org/diseases-conditions/irritable-bowel-syndrome/symptoms-causes/syc-20360016

Irvine, U. of C. (2008, October 10). *How fatty foods curb hunger.* ScienceDaily.

https://www.sciencedaily.com/releases/2008/10/081007123647.htm

Is a food intolerance making weight loss difficult? (2014, May 25). YorkTest. https://www.yorktest.com/us/blog/is-a-food-intolerance-making-it-difficult-for-you-to-lose-weight/

Is inflammation preventing you from losing weight? (n.d.). Dropbio Health. https://www.dropbiohealth.com/health-resources/inflammation-weight-loss

Keys, A., Mienotti, A., Karvonen, M. j., Aravanis, C., Blackburn, H., Buzina, R., Djordjevic, B. S., Dontas, A. S., Fidanza, F., Keys, M. H., Kromhout, D., Nedeljkovic, S., Punsar, S., Seccareccia, F., & Toshima, H. (1986). The diet and 15-year death rate in the seven countries study. *American Journal of Epidemiology*, *124*(6), 903–915. https://doi.org/10.1093/oxfordjournals.aje.a114480

Lawler, M. (2018, August 31). *Celebs who love the keto diet: Kim Kardashian, Halle Berry, and more.* Everyday Health. https://www.everydayhealth.com/ketogenic-diet/diet/celebrities-cant-get-enough-ketogenic-diet/

Lee, C.-Y. S., Goldstein, S. E., Dik, B. J., & Rodas, J. M. (2020). Sources of social support and gender in perceived stress and individual adjustment among Latina/o college-attending emerging adults. *Cultural Diversity and Ethnic Minority Psychology*, *26*(1), 134–147. https://doi.org/10.1037/cdp0000279

Lemos, J. de. (2020, December 16). *Why belly fat is dangerous and how to control it*. UT Southwestern Medical Center. https://utswmed.org/medblog/belly-fat/

LeWine, H. E. (Ed.). (2020, March 25). *How much water should you drink?* Harvard Health. https://www.health.harvard.edu/staying-healthy/how-much-water-should-you-drink

Loy, B. D., O'Connor, P. J., & Dishman, R. K. (2013). The effect of a single bout of exercise on energy and fatigue states: a systematic review and meta-analysis. *Fatigue: Biomedicine, Health & Behavior*, *1*(4), 223–242. https://doi.org/10.1080/21641846.2013.843266

Ludwig, D. S. (2019). The ketogenic diet: Evidence for optimism but high-quality research needed. *The Journal of Nutrition*, *150*(6). https://doi.org/10.1093/jn/nxz308

Mackenzie, M. (2016, September 26). *What your poop can tell you about your belly fat*. Women's Health. https://www.womenshealthmag.com/weight-loss/a19904841/poop-reveals-about-belly-fat/

Madel, R. (2012, April 10). *Exercise as stress relief*. Healthline. https://www.healthline.com/health/heart-disease/exercise-stress-relief#Check-with-Your-Doctor

Mawer, R. (2019, December 15). *A ketogenic diet to lose weight and fight disease*. Healthline. https://www.healthline.com/nutrition/ketogenic-diet-and-weight-loss#What-is-a-ketogenic-diet?

Mensah, G. A., Croft, J. B., & Giles, W. H. (2002). The heart, kidney, and brain as target organs in hypertension. *Cardiology Clinics*, *20*(2), 225–247. https://doi.org/10.1016/s0733-8651(02)00004-8

Meredith, G. R., Rakow, D. A., Eldermire, E. R. B., Madsen, C. G., Shelley, S. P., & Sachs, N. A. (2020). Minimum time dose in nature to positively impact the mental health of college-aged students, and how to measure it: A scoping review. *Frontiers in Psychology*, *10*(2942). https://doi.org/10.3389/fpsyg.2019.02942

Nall, R. (2018, August 17). *How to relieve gas: Easy methods and remedies*. Medical news today. https://www.medicalnewstoday.com/articles/314530

NewBeauty Editors. (2017, May 30). *The "salt depletion" diet this model does before photoshoots is actually really dangerous*. NewBeauty. https://www.newbeauty.com/how-models-prepare-for-photoshoot-salt-depletion

Nikolai Anitchkov, MD. (2006). University of Minnesota. http://www.epi.umn.edu/cvdepi/bio-sketch/anitchkov-nikolai

Nohe, M. (2020, January 22). *Celebrities with food allergies*. Allergy Amulet. https://www.allergyamulet.com/blog/celebrities-with-food-allergies

Obesity and overweight. (2021, June 9). World Health Organization. https://www.who.int/news-room/fact-sheets/detail/obesity-and-overweight

Omega-3 fatty acids. (2019). Cleveland Clinic. https://my.clevelandclinic.org/health/articles/17290-omega-3-fatty-acids

Palinski-Wade, E. (2016, March 26). *Eat fat to reduce belly fat*. For Dummies. https://www.dummies.com/article/body-mind-spirit/physical-health-well-being/diet-nutrition/belly-fat-diet/eat-fat-to-reduce-belly-fat-169518/

Peng, A. W., Juraschek, S. P., Appel, L. J., Miller, E. R., & Mueller, N. T. (2019). Effects of the dash diet and sodium intake on bloating. *The American Journal of Gastroenterology, 114*(7), 1109–1115. https://doi.org/10.14309/ajg.0000000000000283

Petre, A. (2017). *8 foods that can cause constipation*. Healthline.

https://www.healthline.com/nutrition/8-foods-that-cause-constipation

Petre, A. (2020, January 31). *7 foods that can cause constipation*. Healthline. https://www.healthline.com/nutrition/8-foods-that-cause-constipation#3.-Processed-grains

Plowe, K. (2022, March 21). *4 reasons your weight-loss diet is making you gassy, and how to fix it*. Livestrong.com. https://www.livestrong.com/article/271843-why-do-i-have-gas-when-losing-weight

Proctor, L. (2014). The integrative human microbiome project: Dynamic analysis of microbiome-host omics profiles during periods of human health and disease. *Cell Host & Microbe, 16*(3), 276–289. https://doi.org/10.1016/j.chom.2014.08.014

Ruggeri, C. (2016, November 24). *8 Popular foods are responsible for 90+ percent of food allergies*. Dr. Axe. https://draxe.com/health/food-allergy-alternatives/

Symptoms & causes of gas in the digestive tract. (2019, October). National Institute of Diabetes and Digestive and Kidney Diseases. https://www.niddk.nih.gov/health-information/digestive-diseases/gas-digestive-tract/symptoms-causes

Symptoms & causes of gas in the digestive tract. (2023, October 4). National Institute of Diabetes and Digestive and Kidney Diseases.

https://www.niddk.nih.gov/health-information/digestive-diseases/gas-digestive-tract/symptoms-causes

Sachdev, P. (2023, February 26). *High blood pressure symptoms*. WebMD. https://www.webmd.com/hypertension-high-blood-pressure/hypertension-symptoms-high-blood-pressure

Salt and sodium. (2019, May 7). Harvard School of Public Health. https://www.hsph.harvard.edu/nutritionsource/salt-and-sodium/

Salty foods: How sodium affects your weight. (n.d.). Creekside Family Practice. https://www.creeksidefamilypractice.com/blog/salty-foods-how-sodium-affects-your-weight#

Samra, R. A. (2010). *Fats and Satiety* (J.-P. Montmayeur & J. le Coutre, Eds.). PubMed; CRC Press/Taylor & Francis. https://www.ncbi.nlm.nih.gov/books/NBK53550/

Saturated fat. (2021, November 1). American Heart Association. https://www.heart.org/en/healthy-living/healthy-eating/eat-smart/fats/saturated-fats

Smith, J. (2023, April 11). *How to lose water weight: 6 ways*. Medical News today. https://www.medicalnewstoday.com/articles/320603#ways-to-lose-water-weight

Sodium in your diet. (2020). U.S. Food and Drug Administration. https://www.fda.gov/food/nutrition-education-resources-materials/sodium-your-diet

Sodium in your diet use the nutrition facts label and reduce your intake. (2021). U.S. Food and Drug Administration. https://www.fda.gov/media/84261/download

Sodium intake and health. (2019). Centers for Disease Control and Prevention. https://www.cdc.gov/salt/index.htm

Sodium intake for adults and children. (2012). World Health Organization. https://apps.who.int/iris/bitstream/handle/10665/77985/9789241504836_eng.pdf

Solinas, C., Corpino, M., Maccioni, R., & Pelosi, U. (2010). Cow's milk protein allergy. *The Journal of Maternal-Fetal & Neonatal Medicine, 23*(sup3), 76–79. https://doi.org/10.3109/14767058.2010.512103

The power of flat tummy slogans: How they motivate and encourage people. (n.d.). Best Slogans. https://www.bestslogans.com/list-ideas-taglines/flat-tummy-slogans/

13 things diet experts won't tell you about weight loss. (2012, March 19). ABC News. https://abcnews.go.com/Health/diet-secrets-

13-things-experts-weight-loss-good/story?id=15954615

Wade, M. (2015, July 29). *The risks of belly fat*. WebMD. https://www.webmd.com/obesity/features/tAhe-risks-of-belly-fat

Walker-Smith, J. A. (1988). Dietary protein intolerance. *Elsevier EBooks*, 144–184. https://doi.org/10.1016/b978-0-407-01320-9.50011-x

Walters, S. (2018, March 15). *Do you lose weight when you poop? Average weight of poop*. Healthline. https://www.healthline.com/health/do-you-lose-weight-when-you-poop

WebMD Editorial Contributors. (2015, September 24). *What kind of poop do I have?* WebMD. https://www.webmd.com/digestive-disorders/poop-chart-bristol-stool-scale

WebMD Contributors. (2022, November 7). *Testing for food allergies*. WebMD. https://www.webmd.com/allergies/food-allergy-test

WebMD Contributors. (2023, April 25). *Top exercises for belly fat*. WebMD. https://www.webmd.com/fitness-exercise/top-exercises-belly-fat

Wellness & Prevention. (2023, May 30). *Good fats vs. Bad fats*. Scripps Health.

https://www.scripps.org/news_items/4359-good-fats-vs-bad-fats

Westphal, S. A. (2008). Obesity, abdominal obesity, and insulin resistance. *Clinical Cornerstone*, *9*(1), 23–31. https://doi.org/10.1016/s1098-3597(08)60025-3

WHO Media Team. (2023, July 17). *WHO updates guidelines on fats and carbohydrates*. WHO. https://www.who.int/news/item/17-07-2023-who-updates-guidelines-on-fats-and-carbohydrates

Why beans make you fart and how to prevent it. (2023, April 18). Cleveland Clinic. https://health.clevelandclinic.org/why-do-beans-make-you-fart/

Winham, D. M., & Hutchins, A. M. (2011). Perceptions of flatulence from bean consumption among adults in 3 feeding studies. *Nutrition Journal*, *10*(1). https://doi.org/10.1186/1475-2891-10-128

Your digestive system & how it works. (2023a, May 11). National Institute of Diabetes and Digestive and Kidney Diseases. https://www.niddk.nih.gov/health-information/digestive-diseases/digestive-system-how-it-works

Printed in Great Britain
by Amazon